K-12 Schools and Public Health Partnerships

This important book addresses ways that K-12 leaders can develop and maintain partnerships with public health leaders and other community members during times of crises. Drawing on real practices of leaders and insights from public health professionals who helped bring children back into buildings during the COVID-19 pandemic, this book offers clear guidance on how to keep students safe, healthy, and learning during inevitable public health crises that impact K-12 schools. With a focus on building trust, a commitment to equity, and an emphasis on communication, this book highlights the building blocks for successful partnerships. This is a must-have playbook for K-12 and public health leaders on how public health and education can effectively and efficiently partner to respond, recover, and prepare for future crises.

Leah Perkinson is former Director of Strategic Learning & Impact at The Rockefeller Foundation, USA.

Lisa C. Barrios is Director of the Division of Readiness and Response Science at the US Centers for Disease Control and Prevention, USA.

Rebecca Lee Smith is Associate Professor of Epidemiology at the College of Veterinary Medicine and a Health Innovation Professor at the Carle-Illinois College of Medicine at the University of Illinois, Urbana-Champaign, USA.

Rachel Roegman is Associate Professor of Education Policy, Organization, and Leadership at the University of Illinois, Urbana-Champaign, USA.

"Filled with engaging stories and practical solutions to real problems school must solve, *K-12 Schools and Public Health Partnerships: Strategies for Navigating a Crisis with Trust, Equity, and Communication* provides quality research and clear leadership moves. To be proactively prepared for future challenges, read this work and take action. The focus on building trust and effective collaboration is inspiring. Implementing the research-based practices will lead to healthier students and growth in their learning."

— **Jack Baldermann,** *award-winning Superintendent, CUSD 201 - Westmont, IL*

"As a school district administrator during the peak of the COVID-19 pandemic, I witnessed firsthand the daily struggles of ever-changing guidance, limited health expertise, and the profound impact on student learning. Our only path forward was forging partnerships with local and national health organizations—collaborations that reshaped the way schools navigated the crisis and beyond."

— **Anthony Schlorff,** *Associate Executive Director, AASA, The Superintendents Association*

"This cross-cutting book synthesizes lessons learned by K-12 leaders as well as public health advocates who partnered during the COVID-19 pandemic to develop re-opening plans and safely return students and staff into school buildings. The authors construct a framework with the components of trust, equity, and communication; each component is clearly linked with concepts from the leadership and organizational change literature. *K-12 Schools and Public Health Partnerships: Strategies for Navigating a Crisis with Trust, Equity, and Communication* deftly uses this framework to closely document how education-public health partnerships played vital roles in responding to, recovering from, and preparing for crises. As such, this book has relevance and applicability for education and public health leaders as well as for university courses and other training programs seeking to develop individuals' knowledge and skills regarding leading in and through crisis."

— **Sarah L. Woulfin,** *Professor,*
Department of Educational Leadership and Policy,
University of Texas at Austin

"COVID-19 is not the first nor will it be the last public health crisis to challenge our health care and education systems. Hopefully it will be the last where policy is influenced by political misinformation. The approach to the next pandemic must include evidence-based science and a coordinated effort between public health officials and education leaders to ensure no harm is done from both a health and education perspective. This multidisciplinary authored book provides guidance and recommendations that are an essential read in preparation for the next public health crisis."

— **Robert M. Kliegman,** *Professor of Pediatrics,*
Medical College of Wisconsin

K-12 Schools and Public Health Partnerships

Strategies for Navigating a Crisis with Trust, Equity, and Communication

Leah Perkinson, Lisa C. Barrios, Rebecca Lee Smith, and Rachel Roegman

Routledge
Taylor & Francis Group

NEW YORK AND LONDON

Designed cover image: Getty Images

First published 2026
by Routledge
605 Third Avenue, New York, NY 10158

and by Routledge
4 Park Square, Milton Park, Abingdon, Oxon, OX14 4RN

Routledge is an imprint of the Taylor & Francis Group, an informa business

© 2026 Taylor & Francis

The right of Leah Perkinson, Lisa C. Barrios, Rebecca Lee Smith, and Rachel Roegman to be identified as authors of this work has been asserted in accordance with sections 77 and 78 of the Copyright, Designs and Patents Act 1988.

For Product Safety Concerns and Information please contact our EU representative GPSR@taylorandfrancis.com. Taylor & Francis Verlag GmbH, Kaufingerstraße 24, 80331 München, Germany.

Trademark notice: Product or corporate names may be trademarks or registered trademarks, and are used only for identification and explanation without intent to infringe.

K-12 Schools Public Health Partnerships: Strategies for Navigating a Crisis with Trust, Equity, and Communication *was prepared by Dr. Lisa C. Barrios in her personal capacity. The opinions expressed in this book are her own and do not reflect the view of the Centers for Disease Control and Prevention, the Department of Health and Human Services, or the United States government.*

ISBN: 978-1-041-00240-6 (hbk)
ISBN: 978-1-041-00238-3 (pbk)
ISBN: 978-1-003-60884-4 (ebk)

DOI: 10.4324/9781003608844

Typeset in Warnock Pro
by SPi Technologies India Pvt Ltd (Straive)

Access the Support Material: www.routledge.com/9781041002383

Contents

Meet the Author

Leah Perkinson has held more than 30 roles across public health, education, nonprofits, and food service and production. She led national pandemic response efforts, coordinated communities of practice, authored public health guidance, and staffed rape crisis lines. She's delivered healthy relationship programs in K-12, supported process improvements for schools serving students with disabilities, owned a coffee roasting business, baked artisan bread, and coached middle school sports. Her work spans the CDC, The Rockefeller Foundation, Brown University, grassroots organizations, and restaurants. A strategic thinker with blue-collar roots from Philadelphia, Leah brings rigor, grit, and heart to everything she does.

Dr. Lisa C. Barrios has been a leader in the field of school emergency preparedness and response for more than 30 years. Dr. Barrios earned a Doctor of Public Health in health behavior and health education from the University of North Carolina School of Public Health, a Master of Science in behavioral sciences from the Harvard School of Public Health, and a Bachelor of Arts in psychology from the University of Rochester. Across her career, she has led activities to help schools prevent, mitigate, and respond to violence, terrorism, and infectious diseases, including COVID-19. She currently serves as the director of the Division of Readiness and Response Science at the US Centers for Disease Control and Prevention.

Becky Smith is Associate Professor of Epidemiology at the University of Illinois College of Veterinary Medicine and a health innovation professor at the Carle-Illinois College of Medicine. Her research focuses on the surveillance and control of infectious diseases in populations. In this capacity, she has advised on COVID-19 control in a wide variety of settings, including schools and universities, throughout the pandemic. Becky received her DVM and PhD in epidemiology from Cornell University, as well as an MS in biosecurity and risk analysis from Kansas State University.

Rachel Roegman is an Associate Professor of Educational Leadership in the Department of Education Policy, Organization, and Leadership at the University of Illinois, Urbana-Champaign. Her research examines the development and support of equity-focused leaders, with an emerging focus on how to make schools more affirming spaces for transgender and non-binary youth. Rachel's work has been influenced by her experiences as a middle school teacher in traditional and alternative schools and her commitment to anti-racist, equity-focused practice. Her first book, *Equity visits: A new approach to supporting equity-focused school and district leadership* (with David Allen, Larry Leverett, Scott Thompson, and Thomas Hatch, 2019), highlights the need for administrators to examine instruction and equity simultaneously.

Preface

During the COVID-19 pandemic, few institutions were tested as profoundly—or as publicly—as our nation's schools. As K-12 leaders and school staff navigated an unfolding crisis, they worked tirelessly to support student learning, safety, and well-being. What became clear was that schools could not do this work alone. In the midst of a global health emergency, the need for strong partnerships, especially between K-12 and public health leaders, became undeniable.

This book is rooted in that recognition. It draws on what we learned during a time of extraordinary disruption—not to dwell in the past, but to equip leaders for what comes next. By highlighting moments of collaboration, adaptation, and resilience, we aim to codify lessons that can inform future planning—so that the next public health crisis, whatever shape it takes, finds schools better prepared and more connected.

At its core, this book rests on a simple but powerful framework: effective partnerships between K-12 leaders and public health partners are built on trust, equity, and communication. These principles are not just a reflection of what worked—they are a guide for how we prepare, respond, and recover in the future. We hope this framework helps K-12 leaders and public health partners move forward with greater clarity and shared purpose—so that together, they can make life-changing and life-saving decisions during the next public health crisis.

▶ WHAT THIS BOOK IS

This book is a collection of stories and lessons from the field. It documents how districts and public health agencies, despite strained resources and intense pressure, found ways to work together and protect their communities. These examples do not represent every school or district—but they do show what is possible, even under difficult conditions.

We believe cross-sector collaboration is not just helpful—it is essential. When resources are limited, partnerships help districts focus their efforts where they will have the most impact. Not every district starts from the same place. Some have more capacity and stronger infrastructure to respond, or better-aligned local leadership. But we believe every district can start somewhere—and when we start small, we can go big.

K-12 schools already serve as key health infrastructure. They do it through more than 3,900 school-based health centers (School-Based Health Alliance, 2023), nearly 79,000 full-time school nurses (Willgerodt et al., 2024), and the everyday decisions of leaders, educators and staff who prioritize student well-being. This book was written to recognize that work, and to support the partnerships that can make it more effective and more sustainable.

▶ WHAT THIS BOOK IS NOT

This is not a comprehensive chronicle of all those who helped schools reopen, nor does it include every sector or institution involved in pandemic response.

It also does not dive into every variable that shaped school experiences, including cultural and linguistic nuance, or the deep grief and personal sacrifice many educators and health professionals endured. Nor does it examine the unintended harms of mitigation measures, the teacher experience, or persistent challenges that often accelerated alongside the pandemic.

▶ WHY WE WROTE THIS BOOK

We come to this work with over 100 years of combined experience in education and public health—as researchers, professors, public health practitioners, former K-12 teachers, and coaches. During the pandemic, we supported schools and public health agencies across the country, and we found ourselves asking: What helped some partnerships succeed? And more importantly, what can these partnerships teach us about how to lead, adapt, and protect school communities in times of crisis?

In 2022, we had an opportunity to explore these questions. Researchers from the University of Illinois's Urbana-Champaign campus had developed an innovative saliva-based COVID-19 test, and The Rockefeller Foundation funded the team to pilot this test for statewide use in K-12 schools and other settings. When the pilot concluded, program officers and researchers organized a national symposium on lessons learned. We brought together K-12 and public health leaders from around the country to share their work in reopening schools during the pandemic.

Over one and a half days, we hosted 14 panel discussions featuring educators, policymakers, researchers, and public health officials. Keynotes were delivered by national leaders including Dr. Deborah Birx, former White House Coronavirus Response Coordinator under President Trump, and Mary C. Wall, Senior Advisor on the White House COVID-19 Response Team under President Biden. This book reflects what we learned from those conversations, and in the months of work that preceded and followed them.

▶ WHAT WE HOPE THIS BOOK WILL DO

We hope this book will offer practical guidance to K-12 leaders who are still navigating the aftershocks of the pandemic—and those preparing for whatever comes next. We hope it inspires those in public health to see schools as essential partners. And we hope it helps both fields recognize that while we cannot control every condition, we can control how we prepare and whom we work with.

We believe in science-based mitigation strategies, and we believe in the expertise of local leaders. We believe that trust is built over time, that advancing equity requires intentional planning, and that communication is most powerful when it is coordinated and clear.

In a time when public discourse is often shaped by polarization and driven by a vocal minority, we reject the normalization of divisiveness, public shaming, and blame. We believe in the goodness of people, the promise of public education, and the strength of cross-sector partnerships. Most of all, we believe in you—the leaders who continue to show up, adapt, and lead with care.

We hope this book serves not only as a resource but as a reminder: that even in crisis, collaboration is possible—and that through partnership, we can build safer, stronger school communities.

–The Authors

▶ WHO WE WOULD LIKE TO THANK

We offer a heartfelt thank you to public servants, in education and public health, who worked at local, state, and federal levels, to keep all students safe and keep them learning during the pandemic. You have worked 60, 70, 80, 90, even 100 hours a week to keep our school communities in your own backyards and across the country safe. You have made sacrifices as part of your job that you never thought you would have to make. You made high-stakes decisions that had life-changing and life-saving implications. You had your community, your state, your country, and in some cases, friends and family, scrutinizing your every step. You lost colleagues, students, friends, and family members decades before their time. And you found a way to not let the grief, the uncertainty, the pushback, the putdowns, and the politics keep you from doing what needed to get done.

We also thank the more than 250 in-person participants (and even more online), including 95 speakers of the 2022 K-12 COVID-19 Response Across the Country: What Worked, What We Learned, and What's Next Symposium. The framework for partnerships that we present was developed from learning with you during our time together. You represented 39 states, the District of Columbia, and five Tribal Nations. You worked at the local, state, and national level, came from public health, K-12, the private sector, and the non-profit world. This symposium would not have occurred without the amazing support of the University of Illinois Foundations Relations and Special Events Planning teams at the University of Illinois Urbana-Champaign, the University of Illinois System, the Carl R. Woese Institute for Genomic Biology, Brown University School of Public Health and especially Jay Walsh, Vice President for Economic Development and Innovation, who planted the seeds for both the symposium and the book. This book would not be possible without your honest conversations and reflections on your work. Some of you are not able to be publicly named in this book, but we hold your work up anonymously.

We would like to thank the publishing team at Routledge, including the peer reviewers of our book proposal.

We have several colleagues who have supported us in various ways in preparing this book, and we would like to recognize them here. They include Anthony Schlorff, Conghui Huang, Emilie Reagan, Jack Balderrmann, Joni Kolman, Laura Vernikoff, Michael Metivier, Oliver Tapaha, Osly Flores, and Robert Kliegman. While we could not name every person or organization we engaged with, we acknowledge the depth and breadth of contributions from people across the country, many of whom continue this work today.

Many organizations supported the planning and hosting of the 2022 K-12 Symposium in meaningful ways. While there are too many to list here, many are represented by the contributors named in Appendix A. The symposium and subsequent conceptualization of this book were supported in part by a grant from The Rockefeller Foundation.

my eye on the prize. To my DV/SV colleagues, thank you for teaching me to listen first. To UNC-SPH, thank you for showing me what good looks like and how to do more with less. To UVM-MBA program, thank you for teaching me how to do more with more. To Pat Mueller, David Merves, Judy Lee (Evergreen), Mary Brownell (UF), Nicole Gaines (NIMAC), and the team at CAST—thank you for shaping how I think about inclusion and access. Thanks to my co-authors, we're better together. And to my family, my mom, and Me-Me and De-De, thanks for always being there *for me.*

Lisa: I want to thank my many public health colleagues who fight every day to keep the people of the United States, and around the world, safe and healthy, and who step up when there is a public health emergency to do even more. I especially want to acknowledge and thank the CDC's Division of Adolescent and School Health (DASH) for more than *30* years of working with schools to strengthen school-based education, health services, school environments, and community connections. DASH envisions a future where all young people are empowered with the knowledge, skills, and resources to support their health and well-being, and I am honored that this was my mission, too, for more than *25* years. I also want to thank my colleagues on the COVID-*19* emergency response. We worked long days for many months and forged bonds that I expect will last a lifetime. The best part of emergency response is meeting terrific, talented people from across the agency and in the field. Finally, thank you Charlotte, Leo, Norm, and my parents for all of your *support.*

Becky: Many thanks to all the people at University of Illinois who supported, encouraged, and pushed me in the many pivots to my work throughout the pandemic, and to all the members of my research team who were gracious about me being pulled away from mosquitoes, ticks, pigs, and wastewater to think about classrooms and policies. Thank you to my co-authors for their incredible effort and constant focus on what really matters when it comes to school health, and for keeping this work grounded and relevant. And thanks to Alex, Christy, and Ziggy for listening, snuggles, and sing-alongs, all necessary components of my mental *health.*

Rachel: I never imagined I would write about indoor air quality, antigen testing, or school-located vaccinations, so my deepest thanks are for my co-authors and the book contributors who expanded my understandings of K-12 leadership in so many different directions. I did not know what I was saying yes to, when I agreed to our first team meeting, but I am so glad that I did. Thank you to my friends, colleagues, and parents who talked through different parts of this journey. And thank you to Sandi, Serena, and Izzy for supporting my daily word counts, celebrating all the milestones along the way, and encouraging me when I needed it the most. You are *so sigma.*

Foreword

March 13, 2020. It was a Friday. I should have known it would be bad luck.

That was the most fateful school day I experienced as a school district administrator, leading the nation's largest school system through a period of immense upheaval and a public health emergency. Chaos was at our feet with the arrival of SARS-CoV-2 in New York. Just a few short weeks later, there were more than 30,000 cases in the City (and rising rapidly); just about a year later, more than 30,000 of my fellow New Yorkers had been killed by the virus. Our community, families, students, and school employees were shaken, hurting. Everything about the situation felt unprecedented—because it was. We went from our last full day in-person that Friday the 13th, to temporarily calling off in-person operations on March 15th in hopes of reopening weeks later, to transitioning to fully remote learning until the end of the school year on March 23rd, and finally returning full-time in-person across the City on September 21st for the start of the 2020–2021 school year.

Five years on, the return to in-person learning indisputably continues to be my proudest professional achievement. The credit is certainly not all mine to take—the journey and the teams responsible for this unparalleled public sector achievement are a subject worthy of both celebration and study.

For my district, that journey back to in-person learning for all students took about six months, readying a school system of 1.1 million students, 1,600 schools, and about 150,000 staff to safely return to classrooms under exceptional circumstances. We did so through close, intensive coordination between the public school and public health systems of New York City. Under the direction of Mayor Bill de Blasio, city agencies rolled up their sleeves to advance this big, novel project with extraordinary scope—extending our reach to every public employee who affected, and were affected by, the school system, and in close partnership with the labor unions and other key partners. Days were filled with endless calls, "war rooms," building walk-throughs, visits to shipping and receiving facilities, parent town halls and discussions, and much more. At the core of our work was a strong, trusting, cross-functional team comprised of the City's Department of Education and all the hardy public health resources that New York City had to offer—from the City's Department of Health and Mental Hygiene, Health and Hospital System, Department of Buildings, Mayor's Office, and beyond.

In early 2021, I had the extraordinary privilege of taking my experience and expertise to the national stage, serving as senior advisor for school reopening on the White House COVID-19 Response Team under President Joe Biden. That's where I first met two of the best partners anyone could ask for: Dr. Lisa C. Barrios and Leah Perkinson, two of the brilliant authors of this book. From day one, we were in it together—working daily across agencies and in robust engagement with external partners—all united by a shared goal: to break COVID-19's grip on the country and safely return students and staff to in-person learning.

At the White House under President Biden, our job was to coordinate a truly national response—pulling together teams from the U.S. Department of Education, the Centers for Disease Control and Prevention (CDC), the National Institutes of Health, the Food and Drug Administration, the Administration for Strategic Preparedness and Response, and more—making sure every piece of the pandemic fight was strong and connected. Lisa and her CDC colleagues had already built the groundwork for school health guidance; my role was to amplify it, strengthen partnerships to implement it, and make sure the science did not just live in a document, but showed up in practice where it mattered: in schools, safely reopening their doors.

Leveraging the trusted voice of the U.S. Department of Education and partnering with outside organizations to expand our reach, we built a coordinated, national response that moved with urgency, prioritized equity, and translated policy into practice. Working hand in hand with district superintendents and school principals around the country, we helped millions of students—especially those in historically underserved communities—to return to classrooms swiftly and safely, and with the support they needed.

I am incredibly proud of what we built together. Real infrastructure across federal agencies to support a public health response in schools did not exist—but we didn't let that stop us. We moved fast. We stood up major new operations, like launching antigen testing programs and getting $10 billion out the door to support them. We broke down the science for educators, parents, and leaders—everything from hand hygiene to isolation protocols to summer camps and beyond. And we pulled in real partners, like Leah and the team at The Rockefeller Foundation, to extend our reach. Together, we made sure the words we wrote from D.C. and Atlanta didn't just sit on a page—they came alive in real schools, helping leaders implement smart strategies and build better systems for the future.

All told—and under absolutely punishing circumstances—we got the job done. We safely brought America's students and teachers back to school. We prioritized vaccine access for more than six million educators and staff, driving vaccination rates to about 90% by the start of the 2021–22 school year. That same fall, we helped launch nearly 10,000 school-based vaccine clinics for kids ages 5–11, working hand in hand with local, county, and state health and education departments. We built and sustained a nationwide system to deliver free, rapid COVID-19 tests to K-12 schools ultimately distributing more than 140 million tests over the life of the program. And we set up a brand-new internal data system to track COVID-related school closures and mitigation strategies across 100,000 K-12 schools. By fall 2021, almost every school in America was back for full-time, in-person learning—up from less than half of schools just months earlier.

These numbers matter. They represent enormous, historic wins for the public and the institutions serving the public during a time of tremendous uncertainty. These accomplishments are why you should listen closely to the lessons Leah, Becky, Rachel, and Lisa share in this book—because they were right there working with K-12 leaders and public health partners who made these achievements happen.

The writers of these chapters, foreword, and afterword are your colleagues—and together, they distill essential lessons in pandemic preparedness and response that must guide our nation's public health and school systems moving forward.

At the heart of it all is the power of strong, trusting relationships—often built under pressure—to get tough work done. This lesson isn't sector-specific, but it's never been truer than in the partnership between public health and public education during the COVID-19 response. As an educator and district administrator, I saw firsthand how deeply linked I was to my public health counterparts in New York City. The same is true for my work with my federal public health colleagues. It wasn't just the big meetings—it was the day-to-day exchanges, the side conversations, and the moments between the meetings that built the trust and collaboration that made real progress possible. We worked with urgency, fully aware that the fragile progress we made would only hold if we continued to invest in those relationships.

What also sets this group of authors apart was their relentless focus on implementation—making sure every word in a guidance document, a webinar, a website, or even a media interview really meant something in its practical use. What a refreshing change from the usual playbook! This was not an approach of simply stringing together words and walking away; it was a real commitment to seeing things through—from helping leaders write responsible health and safety policies, to getting real dollars and resources (like testing) into schools, and most importantly, staying side-by-side with local leaders to troubleshoot every twist and turn of the public health emergency. The authors' commitment to equity is not just about issuing guidance—it is about making sure that guidance has the greatest chance of *working* for as many schools and students as possible, especially for those at the margins, where the need is greatest. They live out the principle that real equity shows up in the doing, not just the saying.

You should read this book because its central message is essential: we must learn from this moment. The book reflects on what was tested, learned, and debated during the most devastating public health crisis of our time. It offers a practical guide for K-12 leaders on how education and public health can partner effectively to respond to, recover from, and prepare for future emergencies. Drawing on insights from policymakers, scientists, school administrators, and the private sector, it highlights both successful strategies and the unexpected challenges leaders faced. It also outlines the building blocks for strong, sustainable partnerships across K-12 and public health. Throughout the pandemic, education leaders were forced to make critical decisions with incomplete, shifting information in a politicized environment. Even amid the uncertainty, it was clear: reopening schools safely required collaborations built on trust, a commitment to equity, and open and honest communications. I know firsthand: there's no doing this work alone. In New York and in D.C., I leaned hard on trusted colleagues and partners to take on the enormous task of getting schools open safely during COVID-19.

This book's authors were at the center of it all. Advising, problem-solving, lifting up leaders across the country. Always generous with their wisdom, always asking the harder question: how can we do this even better? And just as importantly, how do we make sure more people know how to do it better? That's what they are doing here with this book—sharing the lessons we must carry forward so we are stronger and more ready for whatever comes next.

As discussed in the pages that follow, trust is not built with words; it is built by showing up, over and over, and doing what you said you would do. You'll see this in the examples throughout the book; the authors' commitment to partnership, to action, to getting it right, is real. It was real then, it's real now, and I'd bet anything it'll be real when the next crisis hits, too.

I've returned to the world of leading schools and education systems, but my unexpected detour into public health changed me. The experience left an indelible mark—reshaping not only what I lead, but how I lead. I am a better, stronger leader because of it.

I hope you read this book the way I did—not just absorbing lessons, but feeling a deep sense of partnership and possibility. Because when the next public health challenge hits (and it will), we'll need leaders who don't flinch. We'll need leaders who are ready to face the unknown, so we can unfailingly keep students where they belong: safe, healthy, and engaged in learning at school, every single day. The partnerships we built during the COVID-19 pandemic cannot be discarded, even if we no longer require the same level of intense collaboration that we did in 2020. Instead, it must be adapted to support students' full range of health needs today, while remaining ready to scale up quickly when the next public health crisis emerges. This book is more than a guide—it's a call to action. I hope it helps you find the way forward—and, in doing so, help us all build a future where public health and K-12 education stand stronger than ever, united in purpose, prepared for what lies ahead, and committed to the well-being of every child and community.

Mary C. Wall, Ed.L.D.
Chief of Staff, New York City Department
of Education, 2020–2021
Senior Advisor and Chief of Staff for the Federal COVID-19
Response, The White House, 2021–2023
Deputy Assistant Secretary for P-12 Education, U.S.
Department of Education, 2023–2025

Introduction

The Importance of Partnerships in Times of Crises

1

In the middle of the spring semester, on March 11, 2020, the World Health Organization declared COVID-19 a global pandemic. In response, K–12 students across the United States were sent home, often with little information about when they would return. Some assumed they would be back after one or two weeks. Others were handed laptops, chargers, and packets to tide them over, concerned that the shutdown would be longer. Everyone hoped it would be a short interruption—just a few weeks at home. No one understood how prolonged or disruptive the crisis would become.

But as days turned into months, the uncertainty became disorienting. District leaders had to make rapid decisions about school closures, remote learning plans, staff safety, student meal distribution, and communication with anxious families—all while working with limited information and unclear guidance. Families were suddenly navigating job losses, illness, and childcare challenges, all while supporting children learning from home. Parents, grandparents, older siblings, aunts, and uncles often became de facto teachers. In many households, one adult juggled multiple children's learning schedules—alongside their own jobs, caregiving responsibilities, and the stress of living through a global health emergency. Virtual learning setups varied widely. Some students joined live video calls on laptops

DOI: 10.4324/9781003608844-1

provided by their school districts; others worked on paper packets at kitchen tables. Internet access was uneven. Devices were limited. In most cases, districts had not yet built the infrastructure—or offered the teacher training—needed to make this shift effective (Cashmere, 2020; Varela & Fedynich, 2020).

In the summer of 2020, K-12 leaders and families across the United States faced an impossible set of choices. COVID-19 cases had surged to record highs by July, a second wave was widely expected in the fall and winter, and vaccines were still in development. Teachers worried about their health, their students' learning, and their ability to teach in new formats. Families were divided—some anxious to return to in-person school, and others afraid it was still too dangerous. Reopening schools—or keeping them closed—posed difficult trade-offs, each with potential risks for students, families, and educators. Alongside concerns that schools could accelerate disease transmission, educators, researchers, and policymakers expressed growing concern that extended remote learning would hinder students' academic progress and social-emotional well-being (Dibner et al., 2020). Some experts advocated for a quicker return to classrooms with layered safety measures in place—especially for elementary students—arguing that the academic and developmental benefits outweighed the risks (Dibner et al., 2020). In a time of widespread uncertainty and national unrest, and in states that did not have reopening mandates, local decisions about school reopening were left to district administrators and school boards, and often reflected the values and preferences of individual communities (Collins & Nuamah, 2020; Will, 2020).

IN BRIEF: LAYERED MITIGATION STRATEGIES

Public health agencies have used layered mitigation strategies as a way to prepare for infectious disease threats like the pandemic, based on the idea that multiple strategies be used simultaneously (Qualls et al., 2017). During the COVID-19 pandemic, this approach was popularized as the "Swiss cheese model" (Mackay, 2020, Reason, 1990). Because not every person or institution will follow every strategy and very few strategies are 100% effective, this model illustrates how combining multiple, overlapping safety measures can reduce the spread of COVID-19. Each individual strategy, like hand hygiene, physical distancing, or improved ventilation, is like a single slice of Swiss cheese. On its own, each slice, or layer, has holes—gaps where the virus could slip through. But when stacked together, these slices form a solid barrier, with one layer's strengths covering another's weaknesses. The more layers in place, the stronger the overall defense.

At the start of the fall 2020 semester, roughly 24% of districts resumed fully in-person learning, while 57% remained remote, and 19% adopted hybrid models (Henderson, Peterson, & West, 2021). Importantly, schools were more likely to close, and remain closed longer, in under-resourced communities than in more affluent communities (US ED, 2021a, 2021b). Despite the large numbers of students learning virtually, this modality was not ideal. Teachers who taught virtually struggled to meet the full scope of students' needs. Internet access was inconsistent, district-provided laptops did not always work, and many families had to rely on printed materials. In under-resourced districts, those difficulties were compounded by systemic barriers including housing instability, food insecurity, and fewer adults to support learning.

While some districts quickly deployed mobile hotspots or launched neighborhood learning hubs, these were in the minority. Most districts were not prepared to teach students in virtual environments for extended periods of time. One truth held across districts: students and families were missing what they relied on most from school—daily structure, social connection, emotional support, and consistent opportunities to grow. Research and experience soon confirmed what many educators and families suspected: virtual learning was no replacement for the relationships, routines, and supportive environments that in-person schooling provided (Cortés-Albornoz et al., 2023).

At the same time, virtual learning did not impact all students equally. School closures had a greater impact on lower-income families, those who had a child with a disability, and families with limited or no access to the internet (IES, 2022). Students from these families experienced a greater degree of learning loss than their well-resourced peers (Gee et al., 2023). Additionally,

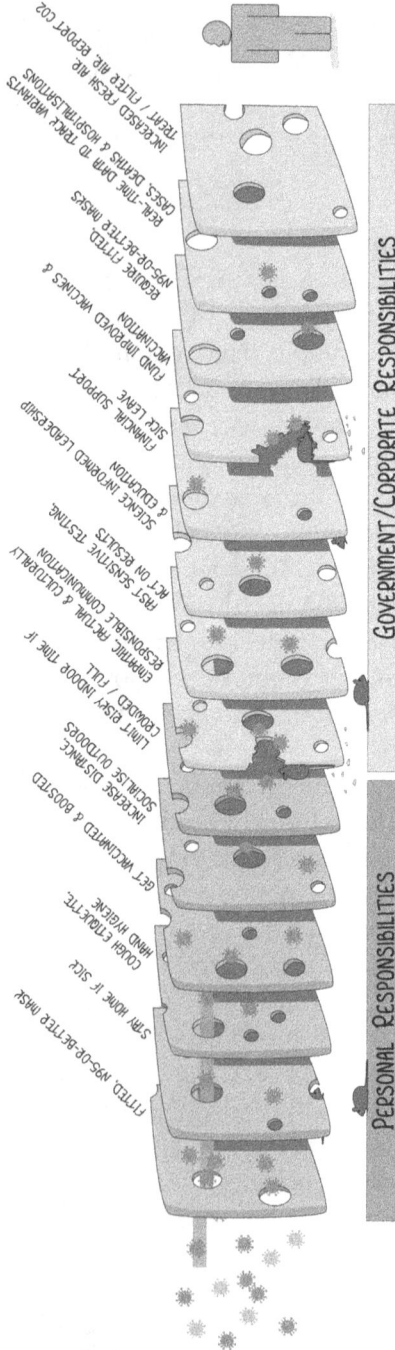

Figure 1.1 The Swiss Cheese Model of Disease Prevention.

parents of children receiving virtual instruction were more likely to experience job loss, reduced work hours, financial and job insecurity, childcare challenges, emotional distress, and difficulty sleeping than those whose children attended school in person (Verlenden et al., 2020).

In addition to facing disruptions to their learning routines and reduced access to classroom instruction, children participating in virtual or hybrid instruction were more likely to experience declines in mental health than those who attended school in person (Verlenden et al., 2020). Over one-third of high school students reported poorer mental health during the pandemic because of disruptions to in-person schooling and relationships with peers and adults; experiences of poorer mental health was especially true for female and lesbian, gay, bisexual, or questioning students (CDC, 2022). For youth living in poverty who relied on school for meals, remote schooling also meant less food when districts were unable to deliver breakfast and lunch (Poole et al., 2021).

Despite concerns with virtual learning, many families of color were wary of returning to in-person learning. Public health data had made clear that COVID-19 compounded health disparities along racial lines (Nana-Sinkam et al., 2021). Long-standing inequities in access to healthcare and higher rates of chronic illness meant that members of communities of color were more likely to experience severe illness or death if they were exposed to the virus. For these families, reopening schools felt less like a return to normal and more like an additional risk—especially in multigenerational households. In these households, older individuals, especially grandparents and great-grandparents, were more at risk of transmission, illness, and hospitalization, and thus, they were more likely to see a return to school as an increase in household exposure. Educators mirrroed this caution: just 35% of teachers of color supported in-person instruction, compared to 47% of White teachers (Will, 2020)—a divide that reflected differing levels of risk and deeper questions about equity, trust, and safety.

By the summer of 2021, it had been more than a year since most U.S. schools first closed their doors. While some schools had resumed in-person instruction earlier, many remained remote or hybrid through much of the 2020–2021 academic year. During that time, districts across the country were preparing for what would become a nearly full return to in-person learning in the fall. It was a pivotal planning moment. In districts large and small, K-12 administrators worked alongside public health partners, community organizations, researchers, and private-sector collaborators to reimagine how schools could reopen safely and equitably. Reopening schools equitably means ensuring that all students have access to appropriate learning opportunities. Doing so required partners to "plan from the margins"—to center students most often pushed to the edges of their communities, because of language, socioeconomic status, or disability, and who were often the most impacted by virtual schooling.

As K-12 leaders across the country moved to in-person learning, they did so within a context of uncertainty. Each week brought new questions with no easy answers: Could ventilation systems be upgraded to reduce airborne transmission? Were distancing protocols feasible in crowded classrooms and narrow hallways? Were there enough working soap dispensers with enough liquid soap to meet basic hygiene needs? Would families choose to send their children back? Leaders were also concerned about staffing shortages, a chronic problem before the pandemic. Bus drivers, nutrition staff, substitute teachers, and school nurses were all in short supply. Some were caring for sick loved ones, others were managing their own health conditions, and many were simply afraid—worried about what returning to school might mean for their safety and the safety of their families. Some districts struggled to keep paper towel dispensers filled, while others worked to retrofit aging HVAC systems in buildings that had not seen capital improvements for decades. The burden on K-12 leaders was immense—balancing public health guidelines, political pressure, community expectations, and the day-to-day needs of students and staff, all while trying to keep schools open and safe.

▶ PARTNERING TO REOPEN

Although COVID-19 was a new disease, K–12 leaders were no strangers to crisis. They were often asked to respond to emergencies with little preparation and limited guidance. Successful crisis management means that leaders engage in evidence-based practices to prepare, prevent, and mitigate events like pandemics or natural disasters (Grissom & Condon, 2021). K-12 leaders knew how to teach through disruption, and they had deep operational expertise and community knowledge. Superintendents and principals understood their district and schools' logistics, staffing realities, and community dynamics. They were used to coordinating transportation, food distribution, and substitute coverage—often across dozens of buildings. They also knew how to translate complex guidance into actionable plans that worked for their students, staff, and families.

At the same time, the pandemic exposed gaps in K-12 leaders' preparedness to respond to a systemic public health emergency. Most school leaders entered the pandemic without formal training on how to coordinate with public health authorities or handle large-scale illness. Their districts lacked the infrastructure, personnel, and protocols to track disease outbreaks, implement evolving safety guidance, or interpret shifting federal recommendations. This is why partnerships with public health leaders—who brought critical tools, data, and health crisis management expertise—were not just helpful, but essential. What began as conversations between schools and public health to understand mask mandates and quarantine rules quickly evolved into deeper collaborations.

This book shares the stories of K-12 and public health leaders who partnered to bring students back into school buildings during the pandemic—and to keep them safe, supported, and learning. During COVID-19, effective school reopenings were driven by K-12 and public health leaders—at local, state, Tribal, and federal levels—who worked in close partnership. While some partnerships existed before the pandemic, many developed through reopening schools together. These collaborations did not happen overnight. They were forged under pressure, often built from scratch, and strengthened by a shared commitment to three core principles: trust, equity, and communication.

This book argues that K-12 and public health leaders cannot afford to let those partnerships dissolve as memories of COVID-19 fade. Instead, they must carry forward what worked, facing the reality that future crises will arise. Grounded in the lived experience of more than 75 K-12 and public health leaders, this book offers a practical framework for cross-sector collaboration—one that can guide preparedness for future public health threats and crises and help ensure schools are ready to respond, recover, and lead.

Throughout this book, we emphasize the importance of K-12 leaders partnering with public health leaders to keep students, staff, and families safe during public health crises. While each field has its own formal definitions for leadership roles, we intentionally broaden those definitions to reflect the realities of cross-sector collaboration. In this book, we define K-12 leaders as those responsible for how schools and districts operate and how students are supported. At the local level, this includes superintendents, principals, school board members, district nurse leaders, special education directors, teacher leaders, and others who have leadership roles during a public health crisis. At the state level, K-12 leaders include state superintendents, members of state boards of education, and others who influence policy, curriculum, funding, and safety decisions that shape schools' ability to respond to public health crises.

We define public health leaders as individuals who shape how communities prepare for, respond to, and recover from public health emergencies. This includes state and local health department directors, Tribal health directors, federal officials at agencies like the Centers for Disease Control and Prevention (CDC), as well as practitioners, policymakers, administrators, scientists, and researchers who design, implement, and evaluate public health strategies. These professionals work across all levels of government, in Tribal health systems, community-based organizations, and academic or policy institutions. Regardless of setting, public health leaders play a central role in ensuring that actions are based in science and informed by evidence-based practices.

▶ PUBLIC HEALTH AT A GLANCE

Public health is the field focused on protecting and improving the health of people and communities. The scope of public health is immense, from clean tap water and restaurant health inspections to new parent workshops and air quality alerts.

Public health professionals promote healthy lifestyles (like encouraging regular physical activity or anti-smoking campaigns), they research disease prevention (such as studying how to reduce the spread of diabetes or heart disease), and they monitor and respond to infectious diseases (like tracking COVID-19 outbreaks or distributing flu vaccines). Unlike doctors and nurses who treat individual patients, public health professionals focus on entire populations. For example, instead of treating someone with lead poisoning, a public health official will ensure that lead pipes in a city's water system are replaced. Their work often involves educational programs (like nutrition classes in schools), research (such as studies on vaccine effectiveness), and policy efforts (like proposing rules to limit sugary drinks in vending machines in schools). Like K-12 education, public health professionals operate at multiple levels—federal, Tribal, state, and local.

The *Centers for Disease Control and Prevention* (CDC) has been a cornerstone of the nation's public health infrastructure since 1946. As the United States' federal public health agency, the CDC issues science-based guidance and best practices to help prevent and control the spread of diseases, promote community health, and protect populations from health threats. During public health emergencies—such as pandemics, natural disasters, or outbreaks—the CDC works with their colleagues at the US Department of Education and other federal agencies to develop guidance that can be used to keep local school communities safe (Kleven et al., 2025). During the pandemic, the CDC developed recommendations for how schools could reduce the spread of COVID-19 based on the best available evidence. While the CDC does not regulate districts, its guidance serves as an important foundation for planning at state, territorial, and local health departments.

As of 2025, the CDC provides funding to local and state public health agencies to support community efforts aimed at preventing and addressing a wide range of health issues. These included chronic diseases like diabetes, infectious diseases like the flu, and preventable injuries and deaths resulting from violence and motor vehicle crashes. The CDC also funds research at academic institutions to better understand the factors that put individuals at increased risk for certain health outcomes and to develop interventions that decrease risk.

The Indian Health Service (IHS) is a federal agency within the US Department of Health and Human Services that provides health services to American Indian and Alaska Native (AI/AN) communities. While not part of the CDC, IHS often collaborates with the CDC and with state and local health departments—especially during public health emergencies—to support disease surveillance, infection control, and vaccination efforts. In school settings, IHS clinics and Tribal health partners may serve as key collaborators for school-based testing, immunization events, or health education programs in Tribal communities.

State and territorial departments of health protect and improve public health across their jurisdictions. They monitor disease outbreaks, manage vaccination programs, regulate health facilities, and oversee statewide public health policies. They also distribute funding to local health departments and help coordinate emergency responses, health communication, and prevention programs.

Local health departments are the front line of public health in communities. They deliver essential services like immunizations, disease surveillance, restaurant inspections, and emergency response. They also communicate directly with the public, support local schools and businesses, and implement health programs tailored to the needs of their populations—often in coordination with state health departments.

▶ A BRIEF HISTORY OF K-12 SCHOOLING DURING PUBLIC HEALTH CRISES

Before COVID-19, public health crises had already shaped K-12 schooling in profound ways. In 1881, the Illinois Department of Public Health required all schoolchildren to be vaccinated against smallpox. In the 1920s, public health and education leaders in New York City partnered to test children for susceptibility to diphtheria and vaccinate them in schools (Brennan-Krohn, 2021). By the 1950s, as polio outbreaks terrified families across the country, school communities played a central role in eradicating the disease by enrolling 1.8 million children in a national vaccine trial. Those trials led to mass school-based vaccination programs the following year, and polio cases dropped by 80% in communities where children were vaccinated (Larsen, 2012). For families, this meant fewer hospitalizations, less time off work, and less fear that everyday childhood activities might result in long-term disability or death.

Today, with modern systems for tracking disease—a practice known in public health as surveillance—decisions during infectious outbreaks in schools often come down to a single, pressing question: *Should schools close, and if so, for how long?* Short-term closures have been shown to slow the spread of viruses like influenza (He et al., 2024), and many educators and families recall facing these decisions during the H1N1 influenza pandemic in 2009.

If you were a K-12 student in 2009, you may have experienced the uncertainty of that moment, especially if you were in a community with an outbreak. In the spring of 2009, as the H1N1 pandemic emerged, the CDC initially recommended school closures of seven days. In response, 726 public schools out of nearly 99,000 across the country temporarily closed (Klaiman et al., 2011). Most closures lasted fewer than seven days and were widely seen as a reasonable tradeoff: a short disruption to prevent broader spread and allow for a quicker return to classrooms. As more data became available, CDC guidance evolved. Blanket closures were no longer recommended, and the agency emphasized that final decisions should be made by local and state officials. In many cases, decisions to close schools were not based solely on infection rates. Instead, they were driven by staffing shortages—when so many educators were out sick that schools simply could not operate safely.

These earlier experiences helped establish some of the routines, relationships, and expectations that shaped how schools would later approach public health more broadly. Most districts were familiar with basic public health practices that prevent the spread of illness—handwashing, covering coughs, staying home when sick, and receiving seasonal flu shots. These measures, grounded in long-standing CDC guidance (Qualls et al., 2017), were typically delivered through partnerships with school nurses, local health departments, school-based wellness programs, or school-based health centers. But not every district had strong ties to public health agencies, and where relationships existed, they tended to focus on routine matters like immunization compliance or health screenings—not emergency response.

When COVID-19 first took hold, school staff relied on what they knew. Teachers reinforced healthy hygiene habits, custodians installed hand washing stations, principals reworked classroom layouts, and nurses fielded parent calls and monitored symptoms. These familiar steps served as the first line of defense in a rapidly evolving crisis before testing, contact tracing (notifying those who have been exposed to the virus), and vaccines became widely available.

But these efforts were not enough. Few districts had plans for large-scale mitigation, widespread testing, or coordinated quarantine protocols (Diliberti et al., 2020). Where school-based health centers (SBHCs) existed, they helped schools coordinate with local health departments—but these centers were not available in every community (School-Based Health Alliance, 2022).

IN BRIEF: SCHOOL-BASED HEALTH CENTERS

The country's 3,900 SBHCs offer access to primary care services as well as a range of other services, potentially including behavioral health, vision, and dental (School-Based Health Alliance, 2022). Working with school health services, SBHCs often serve students who might otherwise lack access to regular healthcare, particularly for children whose families face barriers in accessing care. Reasons for barriers may include lack of sufficient community-based services, family income, or insurance.

▶ THE CASE FOR CONTINUED PARTNERSHIP

By September 2021, nearly all schools (98%) had resumed full-time, in-person learning (National Center for Education Statistics [NCES], 2022). This return marked a major milestone—but it did not signal a return to normal operations. If anything, the challenges were shifting. New variants emerged, and staffing shortages intensified. School facilities were pushed to their limits. Facilities directors worked to retrofit aging HVAC systems in buildings that had not been upgraded for decades. Debates about testing and vaccines spread across communities. New reporting requirements meant that schools had to report COVID-19 test results through outdated school data systems.

Amidst these challenges, leaders faced mounting pressure to keep classrooms open. The months ahead tested not only infrastructure and staffing, but also the resolve of K-12 leaders who made high-stakes decisions under extraordinary, often unprecedented, conditions. In December 2021, the highly transmissible Omicron variant swept across the country, triggering widespread disruptions in in-person learning. By early January, hundreds of schools had temporarily shifted back to remote instruction—not due to high case counts alone, but due to staffing shortages that made it impossible to keep buildings open (Zviedrite et al., 2024).

The lesson was clear: partnerships were a must for keeping students and building staff in K-12 schools safe. K–12 and public health leaders relied on each other's expertise as they responded to evolving guidance, shared timely data, and worked collaboratively to keep students, staff, and families safe.

▶ PARTNERSHIP FRAMEWORK: A SHARED COMMITMENT TO TRUST, EQUITY, AND COMMUNICATION

This book tells the story of how K-12 and public health leaders across the United States came together, over two full years from March 2020 to March 2022, to bring students safely back to school during the COVID-19 pandemic. Drawing from the lived experiences of dozens of leaders in both fields, the chapters that follow document how they responded, adapted, and partnered to meet one of the greatest public health challenges of our time. Using what we learned, we developed a framework to guide the work of building partnerships between K-12 and public health leaders before, during, and after a public health crisis.

Building on our work with K-12 and public health leaders over two years, we convened a national symposium in 2022:

Spring 2020
• National emergency declared
• Schools shift to virtual learning

Spring 2021
• Temporary shifts to virtual learning
• Vaccines become available for children

Spring 2022
• End of public health emergency

Fall 2020
• Testing becomes more available
• Most schools still in virtual learning

Fall 2021
• Most schools return to full-time in-person learning

Figure 1.2 A Brief Timeline of School Reopening.

K-12 COVID-19 Response Across the Country: What Worked, What We Learned, and What's Next. The goal was to elevate on-the-ground voices, reflect on what made cross-sector partnerships successful, and chart a course forward based on the relationships that developed and lessons learned during the first two years of the pandemic. Over the course of a day and a half, 95 speakers from 39 states and the District of Columbia came together, representing education and public health sectors at the community, state, Tribal, and federal levels. They shared how they launched, sustained, and strengthened school–public health partnerships during the pandemic.

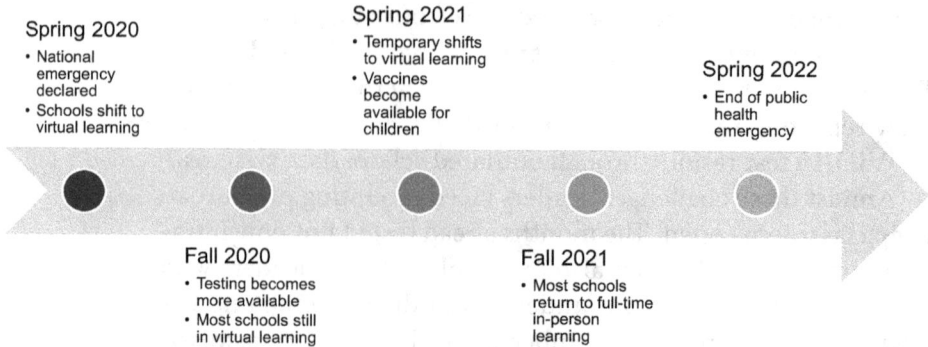

To assemble this body, we began by inviting speakers from the Cross-City Learning Group (CCLG), a community of practice convened by one of this book's authors at The Rockefeller Foundation, Leah Perkinson. In addition to members of the CCLG, we also invited K-12 and public health experts from our professional networks to share their experiences and help us to define a set of topics on which to focus the symposium's sessions.

IN BRIEF: THE CROSS-CITY LEARNING GROUP (CCLG)

The CCLG was a peer network of K-12 and public health leaders convened by The Rockefeller Foundation. The group had three goals:

1. to provide technical support to districts and their public health partners as they established school-based testing programs;

2. to facilitate problem-solving and resource sharing across diverse contexts; and
3. to surface promising practices and lessons learned to inform a national K-12 testing playbook for districts and their public health partners across the country.

Created to support school- and community-based COVID-19 testing at the height of the pandemic, the CCLG emerged during a period of deep uncertainty and urgent need. The group brought together about 30 leaders from school districts and public health departments across the country, university researchers, diagnostic experts, and a senior advisor to the mayor of a major US city. It was a space for rapid learning, candid exchange, and collaborative problem solving—the kind of partnership this book seeks to highlight. Over the course of one year, beginning in fall 2020, CCLG members met weekly—sometimes twice a week—to learn about each other's testing programs in real time.

We developed this framework for partnerships based on our learnings from K-12 and public health leaders who presented at the symposium and many follow-up conversations afterward. At the heart of this book is a simple but powerful idea: effective K-12 and public health partnerships rest on three interdependent principles: **trust**, **equity**, and **communication**. A commitment to building and earning *trust*—between individuals and between institutions—is the foundation of any coordinated response. Without it, collaboration breaks down; with it, partnerships are strengthened and more resilient in the face of uncertainty. A commitment to *equity* means more than the pursuit of fairness—it requires deliberately reaching and including those most likely to be overlooked, underserved, or excluded. In public health emergencies, planning from the margins ensures that these individuals, the students and families with least access, are not an afterthought but a starting point. A commitment to *communication* means a shared agreement and multidirectional approach to developing clear, fact-based messages that flow between institutions and stakeholder groups.

These principles are not abstract ideals. During the pandemic, they became shared commitments that translated into concrete strategies, guiding leaders at every level. From district

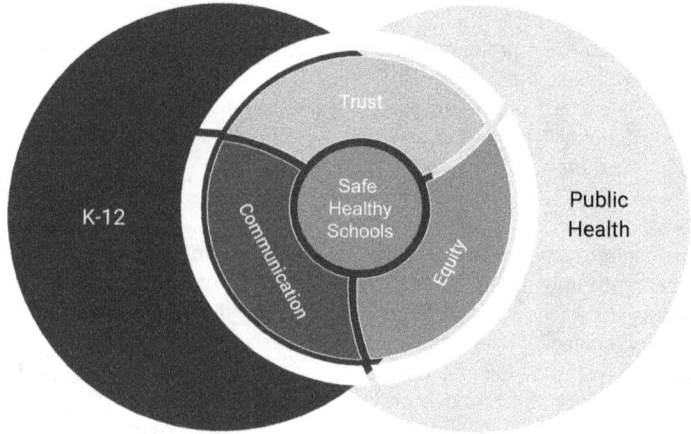

Figure 1.3 Partnership Framework: A Shared Commitment to Trust, Equity, and Effective Communication.

nurse leaders to state superintendents, and from community health workers to state health directors, these principles helped K-12 and public health leaders work effectively to keep students safe as buildings reopened. In the chapters that follow, we examine how each principle—trust, equity, and communication—showed up in practice, shaped decisions, and offered a path forward.

▶ WHAT TO EXPECT IN THE CHAPTERS AHEAD

In the chapters that follow, we explore the three principles that underpin our framework for effective K-12–public health partnerships. Each chapter focuses on one principle in depth. We begin by introducing the principle and describing its key features. We share examples and reflections from partners that illustrate how these features play out in practice, often overlapping with and reinforcing the others. Each chapter also includes a detailed case example that highlights how the principle takes shape over time in practice. We conclude with concrete steps that K-12 and public health leaders can use to build or strengthen partnerships in their own communities—not just during emergencies, but during everyday planning and decision-making.

In Chapter 2, we explore how K–12 and public health leaders built and sustained trust during the pandemic. We begin by examining the defining features of *relational trust*—the personal interactions and behaviors that foster confidence between individuals, including respect, personal regard, competence, and integrity—and how partners demonstrated these in their day-to-day collaboration. We then turn to *institutional trust* and highlight how organizations earned credibility by serving others, demonstrating reliability, and aligning with community values.

This chapter continues with a case study from Birmingham, Alabama, illustrating how K-12 and public health leaders worked together to rebuild trust in communities where public health systems had once caused harm. In a city shaped by a long history of racial inequity—including painful periods when Black communities were excluded from decision-making or subjected to unethical medical practices—this work was both urgent and deeply personal.

In Chapter 3, we explore what it means to plan from the margins as a way to think about equity. This chapter highlights how K-12 and public health partners worked to define and pursue equitable academic and health outcomes during the pandemic. Key strategies include using both prioritization—identifying who needs which supports first—and differentiation—adapting supports to reflect the specific needs and strengths of students, staff, and families.

In this chapter, our case is set in Louisville, KY against the backdrop of Jefferson County Public Schools' long-standing commitment to racial equity. The case illustrates how district and public health leaders worked together to pursue equitable outcomes on three levels: for individual students and families, across school buildings, and districtwide. We also explore how the district-wide racial equity policy shaped reopening decision-making and supported students' return—not just to classrooms, but to safe, stable, and nurturing environments.

In Chapter 4, we explore the concept of communication. We identify central practices related to effective communication, including the role of trusted messengers and the importance of multidirectionality and transparency. We also address ways to respond to inaccurate health information.

This chapter's case explores how one district, Aurora Public Schools in Colorado, used clear, multilingual, and family-centered communication to build trust, align with public health partners, and keep students learning safely in person. The district prioritized frequent, multilingual messaging that was consistent, inclusive, and responsive to family concerns. This steady communication helped build trust and foster a sense of partnership between families who spoke languages other than English and district personnel.

In the concluding chapter, we bring the lessons together and we reflect on what partnerships reveal about the broader role of schools and K-12 leaders during a public health crisis. In this sense, we look back to move ahead, drawing on what we learned to support what we can do now. We argue that when K-12 leaders and communities adopt a public health mindset, they recognize schools' critical role in keeping students and staff safe and how building and sustaining partnerships with public health leaders strengthens that role. We end with a final set of recommendations for partnership work and remind everyone that by committing to partnership, we can ensure that schools remain safe places where all students can learn—no matter what crises the future brings.

We also include a set of appendices with brief biographies of the leaders who contributed to this work (Appendix A), a teaching guide for university classrooms (Appendix B), a curated resource list for more reading on various topics across the book (Appendix C), a list of commonly used abbreviations from K-12 and public health (Appendix D), tips for creating a community survey (Appendix E), and a guide for developing a data dashboard (Appendix F).

The pandemic made clear that schools are more than places where students go to learn—they are communities within communities that offer meals, health care, mental health support, and more. These functions are strongest when K-12 and public health leaders work hand in hand.

Across the country, we have seen that when K-12 and public health leaders commit to building partnerships rooted in trust, centered on equity, and guided by communication, they strengthen relationships and deliver more effective responses. When these principles anchor the work, leaders are better prepared to navigate public health crises—before, during, and after they occur.

This book is not just about COVID-19. It is a book about what the pandemic taught us about building strong, lasting partnerships between schools and public health agencies. These lessons are not confined to the past. They are meant to be applied now, and in the future. What we do now—how we plan, build trust, and strengthen relationships—will shape how ready we are to protect students, support families, and keep schools open and safe when the next moment comes. By looking back together, we hope to help leaders move forward equipped with stronger partnerships, practical tools, and a clearer understanding of what it takes to keep students healthy, safe, and learning.

References

Brennan-Krohn, T. (2021). *Making school safe during outbreaks: Diphtheria and COVID-19.* American Society for Microbiology. Retrieved from https://asm.org/articles/2021/september/making-school-safe-during-outbreaks-diphtheria-and

Cashmere, D. J. (2020). Teachers turn to crowdfunding for pandemic supplies. Marketplace. Retrieved from https://www.marketplace.org/2020/10/02/teachers-crowdfunding-pandemic-supplies-remote-learning-equipment/

Centers for Disease Control and Prevention. (2022). Youth Risk Behavior Survey Data Summary and Trends Report: 2011–2021. Atlanta, GA; US Department of Health and Human Services. Retrieved from https://www.cdc.gov/yrbs/dstr/index.html

Collins, J. E., & Nuamah, S. A. (2020). Americans overwhelmingly oppose school reopenings, data finds. *Washington Post*, August 19, 2020. Retrieved from https://www.washingtonpost.com/politics/2020/08/19/americans-overwhelmingly-oppose-school-reopenings-new-data-finds/

Cortés-Albornoz, M. C., Ramírez-Guerrero, S., García-Guáqueta, D. P., Vélez-Van-Meerbeke, A., & Talero-Gutiérrez, C. (2023). Effects of remote learning during COVID-19 lockdown on children's learning abilities and school performance: A systematic review. *International Journal of Educational Development, 101*, 102835.

Dibner, K. A., Schweingruber, H. A., & Christakis, D. A. (2020). Reopening K-12 schools during the COVID-19 pandemic: A report from the National Academies of Sciences, Engineering, and Medicine. *JAMA, 324*(9), 833–834.

Diliberti, M., Schwartz, H. L., Hamilton, L. S., & Kaufman, J. H. (2020). Prepared for a Pandemic? How Schools' Preparedness Related to Their Remote Instruction during COVID-19. Data Note: Insights from the American Educator Panels. Research Report. RR-A168-3. *Rand Corporation.*

Gee, K. A., Asmundson, V., & Vang, T. (2023). Educational impacts of the COVID-19 pandemic in the United States: Inequities by race, ethnicity, and socioeconomic status. *Current Opinion in Psychology, 52*, 101643.

Grissom, J. A., & Condon, L. (2021). Leading schools and districts in times of crisis. *Educational Researcher, 50*(5), 315–324.

He, C., Norton, D., Temte, J. L., Barlow, S., Goss, M., Temte, E., Bell, C., Chen, G., & Uzicanin, A. (2024). Effect of planned school breaks on student absenteeism due to influenza-like illness in school aged children: Oregon School District, Wisconsin September 2014–June 2019. *Influenza and Other Respiratory Viruses, 18*(1), e13244.

Henderson, M. B., Peterson, P. E., & West, M. R. (2021). Pandemic parent survey finds perverse pattern: Students are more likely to be attending school in person where covid is spreading more rapidly. *Education Next, 21*(2), 34–49.

Institute of Education Sciences. (2022). Digest of Education Statistics, 2020. Retrieved from https://ies.ed.gov/use-work/resource-library/report/compendium/digest-education-statistics-2020

Klaiman, T., Kraemer, J. D., & Stoto, M. A. (2011). Variability in school closure decisions in response to 2009 H1N1: A qualitative systems improvement analysis. *BMC Public Health, 11*, 1–10.

Kleven, D., Barrios, L. C., Fineman, L., Kanade Cramer, N., & Roy, W. (2025, June 16). School-related public inquiries received by the

Centers for Disease Control and Prevention during the COVID-19 pandemic, United States, 2020–2022. medRxiv. https://doi.org/10.1101/2025.06.16.25329578

Larsen, D. (2012). The march of dimes and polio: Lessons in vaccine advocacy for health educators. *American Journal of Health Education, 43*(1), 47–54.

Mackay, I. M. (2020). The swiss cheese respiratory virus defense. Figshare Figure. https://doi.org/10.6084/m9.figshare.13082618.v26

Nana-Sinkam, P., Kraschnewski, J., Sacco, R., Chavez, J., Fouad, M., Gal, T., ... & Behar-Zusman, V. (2021). Health disparities and equity in the era of COVID-19. *Journal of Clinical and Translational Science, 5*(1), e99.

National Center for Education Statistics. (2022). *Impact of the COVID-19 pandemic on elementary and secondary education.* U.S. Department of Education, Institute of Education Sciences. https://nces.ed.gov/surveys/annualreports/topical-studies/covid/

Poole, M. K., Fleischhacker, S. E., & Bleich, S. N. (2021). Addressing child hunger when school is closed: Considerations during the pandemic and beyond. *New England Journal of Medicine, 384*(10), e35.

Qualls, N. L., Levitt, A. M., & Kanade, N. Qualls, N. (2017). *Community mitigation guidelines to prevent pandemic influenza—United States, 2017. MMWR.* Recommendations and reports, 66.

Reason, J. (1990). *Human error.* New York: Cambridge University Press.

School-Based Health Alliance. (2022). *The School-Based Health Alliance children's health and education mapping tool.* Washington, DC: School-Based Health Alliance. https://data.sbh4all.org/sbhadb/maps/

U.S. Department of Education (2021a). Institute of Education Sciences, National Center for Education Statistics, School Pulse Panel, July-September 2021. Retrieved from https://nces.ed.gov/surveys/annualreports/topical-studies/covid/theme/elementary-and-secondary-education-shifts-in-enrollment-and-instructional-mode/

U.S. Department of Education. (2021b). Institute of Education Sciences, National Center for Education Statistics, Monthly School Survey, 2020–21 school year. Retrieved from https://ies.ed.gov/schoolsurvey/mss-dashboard/

Varela, D. G., & Fedynich, L. (2020). Leading schools from a social distance: Surveying south texas school district leadership during the COVID-19 pandemic. *National Forum of Educational Administration and Supervision Journal, 38*(4), 1–10.

Verlenden, J. V., Pampati, S., Rasberry, C. N., et al. (2020). Association of children's mode of school instruction with child and parent experiences and well-being during the COVID-19 pandemic—COVID Experiences Survey, United States, October 8–November 13, 2020. *MMWR. Morbidity and mortality weekly report, 70.*

Will, M. (2020). Most teachers don't want in-person instruction, fear COVID-19 health risks. *Education Week.* Retrieved from https://www.edweek.org/leadership/surveys-most-teachers-dont-want-in-person-instruction-fear-covid-19-heath-risks/2020/07

Zviedrite, N., Jahan, F., Moreland, S., Ahmed, F., & Uzicanin, A. (2024). COVID-19–related school closures, United States, July 27, 2020–June 30, 2022. *Emerging Infectious Diseases, 30*(1), 58.

Building and Maintaining Trust

> We've had a long-standing partnership with the University of Wisconsin to fight the flu—and that foundation mattered when COVID hit. One of the lead researchers lives just a block from our school. Families know him. We know the people in his lab. There's a lot of trust built up over the years, and that trust made all the difference. It helped people feel more at ease when we began testing for COVID.
>
> Dr. Leslie Bergstrom, Superintendent,
> Oregon School District, Wisconsin

In early 2021, there was a strong push to re-open K-12 school buildings. K-12 and public health leaders across the country needed to develop and implement plans that families and educators trusted would keep them safe. For Dr. Bergstrom, superintendent of a seven-school, 4,000-student district south of Madison, Wisconsin, preexisting trust between the district, the community, the local university, and public health agencies was key to enabling in-person schooling for all students by Spring 2021, less than one year after schools across the country closed. District leaders worked with their partners to implement COVID-19 mitigation strategies as students returned to the building. Broad acceptance and uptake of these recommended strategies was due, in part, to the trust the

DOI: 10.4324/9781003608844-2

school community had in the individuals and institutions behind the recommendations.

This chapter explores the dimensions of trust that enabled K-12 and public health leaders across the country to plan reopening strategies and welcome students back into schools. We examine trust at two levels: the trust between individuals and the trust placed in institutions or systems. *Relational trust*—the confidence one person places in another—can often serve as a gateway to *institutional trust*—the belief that an organization is competent, caring, and ethical. When someone consistently acts with competence, integrity, and care, they not only establish personal credibility but also reinforce trust in the school, district, or public health department they represent.

We then turn to Birmingham, Alabama, where leaders from the University of Alabama at Birmingham and Birmingham City Schools worked to strengthen trust in public health efforts—asking families to place their faith in tools and guidance issued by systems that, in the past, had failed to protect them. This case shows that while trust cannot be rebuilt overnight, creating space for honest dialogue and leading with empathy can begin to repair relationships and restore public confidence in public health recommendations. We close the chapter with practical considerations for K–12 and public health leaders seeking to build, repair, and maintain trust—especially when time is limited and the stakes are high.

▶ WHAT TRUST IS AND HOW IT DEVELOPS

Trust is the belief that a person—or an institution, organization, school, or district—is reliable, competent, and acting in good faith. People do not trust someone because they are in a position of authority, but because that person can be counted on, cares about their well-being, and has the expertise to do their job well. During the pandemic, K-12 and public health leaders had to earn trust from each other and from community stakeholders quickly, often under intense pressure.

REFLECTIONS FROM THE FIELD: IN PARTNERSHIP, THE FIRST COMPONENT IS TRUST

Mara G. Aspinall worked as an advisor to The Rockefeller Foundation during the pandemic, co-founded the Biomedical Diagnostics program at Arizona State University, and was a key technical advisor for the CCLG. She shares a key lesson learned from her work helping districts to implement testing programs.

All involved, but especially the school administrators, needed to be creative and flexible. Schools were not organized to do disease testing, and they needed to be creative to find solutions that would work and still conduct the learning necessary for the school's primary function. To make testing happen, the first component was building trust to and from all constituencies. Trust needed to be established within a school district: between parents and administrators, between administrators and teachers and staff, as well as between administrators and students. Trust also needed to be established between the district and the state or federal agency managing the allocated monies. Lastly, trust with the testing company was essential. Without all this trust, programs were not embraced and therefore not effective.

When trust exists prior to a crisis, it allows people to move forward together and can lead to better outcomes, such as participation rates in testing programs, as shared by Rhiannon Walker, former school nurse with the Whiteriver Unified School District, serving about 2300 students in Arizona. Walker was responsible for enrolling students in the district's testing program. "One way I was able to obtain consent was the relationship that I already had with the community. I knew my students and their families. I was able explain how the testing worked and why we were doing it." Trusted relationships and meeting with families face to face led to increased participation in Whiteriver's testing program. Dr. Sonia Lee, Branch Chief at the Eunice Kennedy Shriver National Institute of Child Health and Human Development agreed that prior connections were essential. She reflected that "We were able to build upon the foundation of trust and partnership to achieve results."

While it is ideal to build trust before an emergency, it can also be built during the response—shaped by how leaders engage, communicate, and act under pressure. Dr. Kanecia Obie Zimmermann, associate professor of Pediatrics at Duke University in Durham, North Carolina, reflected on how she developed trust with different stakeholders during the pandemic. She was "willing to meet people where they were; and pursued answers to questions that benefited partners, not just the questions my team was interested in." Her approach captures the essence of trust—meeting partners where they are and pursuing answers that matter to them—a theme that carries through the next sections as we explore both relational and institutional trust in action. In the sections that follow, we outline the defining dimensions of relational trust, then turn to institutional trust—using real-world examples to illustrate how each takes shape and why both matter in times of crisis.

Relational Trust and Its Defining Dimensions

Trust is a central requirement for effective partnerships. Research on school improvement consistently emphasizes that successful schools are grounded in trust: between educators and administrators, and between schools and the students, families, and communities they serve (Bryk and Schneider, 2003; Hallam & Hausman, 2009; Louis, 2007). In times of uncertainty requiring high-stakes decision-making, trust helps individuals, communities, and organizations move forward together. Ideally, trust is already strong across all levels prior to a public health crisis—but it can also grow during the response.

Bryk and Schneider (2003) spent four years studying more than 400 elementary schools in Chicago. Through this research, they defined relational trust as "an interrelated set of mutual dependencies [that] are embedded within the social exchanges in any school community" (p. 41). These mutual dependencies take shape as teachers, administrators, students, and families rely on one another to fulfill shared responsibilities—such as creating safe, welcoming schools and maintaining high expectations for learning and collaboration. Trust grows when people consistently

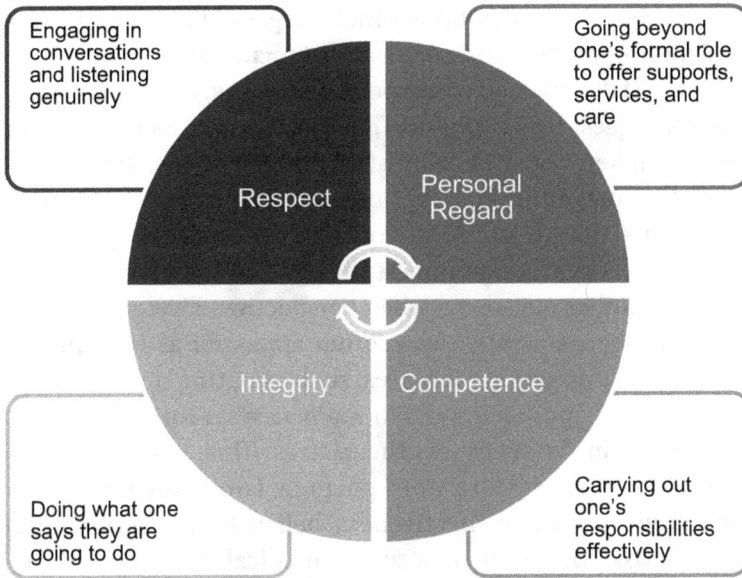

Figure 2.1 Elements of Relational Trust (Bryk & Schneider, 2003).

follow through on their commitments, showing others that they can be relied upon over time.

Bryk and Schneider (2003) argue that there are four key dimensions that make up relational trust: (1) respect, (2) personal regard for others, (3) competence, and (4) integrity. Together these dimensions contribute to how much trust one person extends to another. We discuss these dimensions in order next, with the understanding that high levels of trust are most likely to occur when all four are present in everyday interactions.

Respect

Respect is expressed when someone listens—especially in moments of disagreement—demonstrating that they value others' perspectives, honor their voice, and recognize their dignity. During the pandemic, as tensions rose over how and when to reopen schools, K–12 and public health leaders had to listen carefully across lines of disagreement. Decisions about mitigation strategies were rarely simple. Leaders had to weigh competing concerns and a wide range of options—including masking, vaccinating, ventilation upgrades, and physical distancing. (Physical distancing was initially referred to as social distancing, but public health agencies suggest using "physical", because using "social" unintentionally implied not socializing at all, instead of socializing safely (Pandi-Perumal et al., 2021)). However, respect as a key dimension means that trust does not require uniform agreement. Instead, it grows through honest dialogue and the willingness to hear one another out—even when perspectives diverge.

During the pandemic, what often appeared as hesitancy or resistance to mitigation measures, such as opting out or taking a "wait and see" approach, was, in many cases, more accurately a lack of trust in the measures themselves. This was shaped by a range of factors: pressure from peers or family members, concerns about safety and effectiveness, beliefs that infection posed minimal risk, beliefs in inaccurate medical information, or a reluctance to follow guidance from institutions or individuals who lacked credibility in the eyes of the community. In these instances, respectful listening became a critical leadership skill. When parents, students, and educators felt that their concerns were acknowledged, they felt respected—and that sense of respect often laid the groundwork for trusting recommendations from public health agencies or officials. Similarly, by intentionally "listening before leading," Dr. Anne Wyllie and her team at the Yale School of Public Health built the trust that helped make widespread participation in school-based COVID-19 testing possible. Wyllie emphasized that trust was earned not through scientific innovation, but through the deliberate act of creating space to hear community concerns, and using those concerns to inform decisions. Her development of a saliva-based COVID-19 test—and her team's national effort to expand test access—succeeded in part because they prioritized listening as a foundation for partnership.

A similar approach guided Jessica Kjar, former COVID-19 K-12 school testing program manager at the Utah Department of Health and Human Services. As she worked to implement school-based testing statewide, she made time to listen to those doing the work on the ground. "We talked with school leaders and local health departments about testing," Kjar explained. "We valued what they had to say, and we wanted them to know that their perspectives were heard and genuinely respected. We adapted programs based on what they could offer and what they needed." Respectful listening led to increased trust between local and state leaders, which ultimately led to an increase in school-based testing programs.

Respect also includes recognizing and honoring individuals' autonomy, or their right to make informed decisions about their own health. This is also a core principle of medical ethics (Gillon, 2003). Enabling community members to make their own decisions about participating in mitigation measures was not just strategic. In states that did not have any mitigation mandates, this approach was required. One state public health official described their approach as "very much person- and people-empowered. People in our state would not want to be told what to do." In these settings, and in partnership with local districts, states offered voluntary testing, used off-site locations to reduce pressure on schools, and shared case rate data regularly to support informed, autonomous decision-making. When leaders offer clear information, meaningful choices, and space for concerns to be voiced, they demonstrate respect by affirming each person's right and capacity to make informed decisions.

Transparent data sharing also creates an opportunity for leaders to show respect and trust in stakeholders, while enabling them to make choices based on the most current information at the time. Brittany Layman, Director of Health, Wellness, and Safety at Regional School Unit 22 in Hampden, Maine with about 2300 students, described how her district worked to keep the school community informed and engaged once state mandates were lifted. Her team developed a public-facing dashboard that reported how many COVID-19 tests had been conducted and how many returned positive, giving families a clear view of where the virus was spreading and how quickly. "The community needed to understand why this work mattered," Layman reflected.

As school nurses, we had a responsibility not just to protect student health, but to keep families informed. By being transparent, showing our confidence in the data, and engaging the community every step of the way, we earned their trust—and they came right along with us.

REFLECTIONS FROM THE FIELD: BUILDING TRUST ACROSS DIFFERENCES

Respect does not always mean agreement. For Joel Solomon, Senior Program Manager, Health and Safety, with the National Education Association, a union of over 3 million members, trust was important in advancing student learning, despite often strong disagreements.

> In confronting COVID-19, the National Education Association worked in national, state, and local contexts in which varying degrees of trust existed before the pandemic. We saw from the beginning of COVID that consensus and acquiescence were not—and did not need to be—synonymous with trust. Instead, even when we disagreed over policies, procedures, and actions to deal with the pandemic and its impact, sharing the practical and technical knowledge and experience of educators of all types, even when we had to insist on being heard, led to better outcomes, the identification of common interests, and greater trust.

Personal Regard

Personal regard is the dimension of relational trust that reflects people going beyond their official roles to support the well-being of others. Leaders show this when they take action not because they have to, but because they choose to. During the pandemic, personal regard showed up in powerful and varied ways. Local superintendents staffed drive-through testing sites, state superintendents drove moving trucks loaded with test kits across the state, principals joined school-wide cleaning routines, and school nurses met one-on-one with families to get input on proposed reopening plans. Trust often grew from small, steady gestures that demonstrate personal regard: a check-in, a helping hand, a willingness to go the extra mile. In Alachua County, Florida, that willingness looked like knocking on doors.

In Alachua County Public Schools (~30,000 students) María Virginia Giani and her team didn't stop at phone calls or emails when attendance dropped. "We did our outreach in waves," Giani explained. "As part of the first wave, we left door hangers on front doors. But students still didn't come. So, we moved on to the second wave-teams going door to door, just talking with students and families to see what was happening."

Giani remembered that families were surprised to see them—but eager to talk. "They wanted to share why they hadn't come back, what movie they had seen last week, how their friends at school were doing," she said. "It meant a lot to them to see us show up like that."

That same spirit of care shaped the response at Chief Leschi Schools (CLS), a Tribally Controlled School (TCS) of 650 students in Washington State operated by the Puyallup Tribe the spuyaləpabš (Puyallup Tribe of Indians, n.d.). A TCS is a school that is contracted with and funded by the Bureau of Indian Affairs, but that is operated by a federally recognized Tribe. As schools closed in the spring of 2020, CLS staff quickly mobilized to keep students connected. They used federal relief funds to purchase laptops and Wi-Fi hotspots for all 650 students. They organized a drive-through dinner where families received food, then stayed in their cars while masked staff provided one-on-one support to set up devices and log in. These efforts reflected a deep sense of personal regard for families, rooted in care, respect, and the belief that every student mattered.

This kind of regard was not always grand or technical—it was often demonstrated by simply "showing up and keeping showing up." For Dr. Jason Newland, who worked at Washington University during the pandemic, "that meant being physically present—visiting communities on their terms, in their spaces. Going the extra mile and getting out of your comfort zone so they can stay in theirs." Newland also reflected on what it meant to "show up" as himself. A pediatrician and community health leader, he initially drew on his professional identity when he presented at community meetings. But colleagues Cynthia Williams and Dr. Sheretta Butler-Barnes encouraged him to let go of the "doctor hat." "You just need to be yourself," they told him. When Newland began sharing more about his own life—talking about his family, his hobbies, and asking others about theirs—something shifted. He was no longer seen as just a doctor, but as a person who genuinely cared about the community. That same ethic of relational care guided the work of his colleague, Butler-Barnes, who emphasized finding "simple ways to sustain relationships," pointing to acts like sending a check-in email or a holiday card or bringing a colleague their favorite coffee drink. Small gestures can carry enormous weight. They signal respect, reliability, and care.

Demonstrating personal regard is rarely a one-time event. It often becomes visible over time, as individuals accumulate opportunities to demonstrate that they have others' best interests at heart. As Dr. Mary C. Wall, former senior advisor and chief of staff for the Federal COVID-19 Response, explained, personal regard is something that "shows up in the moments between the meetings." For Ashley Hill, associate director of the State and Territory Alliance for Testing, this dimension can be summed up even more simply, in one word: kindness. Working alongside public health leaders across the country during the pandemic, she saw just how much trust mattered—and how quickly it could be built, even under pressure. For Hill, it came down to one thing:

> Believing in the power of kindness and being helpful. Everyone is doing their best under pressure, and how you show up can make a real difference. Being kind builds trust quickly and creates a more collaborative environment. In crisis response, trust is everything—and a little kindness goes a long way in helping teams stay focused and move forward together.

The importance of kindness was reinforced by Sarah Sutton, former director of school programs at Health Commons, a Washington-based nonprofit organization that provided technical assistance for district leaders through a community of practice (COP). Communities of practice are formal or informal groups of practitioners who work together to solve problems in specific focus areas (Wenger, 1998). Sutton and her team earned the trust of districts by focusing on offering practical help. "We found we could build trust just by making one thing easier for them," she recalled. "That's what kept members of the COP coming back."

IN BRIEF: STATE AND TERRITORY ALLIANCE FOR TESTING (THE STAT NETWORK OR STAT)

In August 2020, six governors met to brainstorm ways to use their states' purchasing power to address shortages in COVID testing supplies. State officials from these six states created the STAT Network, an action network launched by The Rockefeller Foundation and sustained by Brown University's School of Public Health. The STAT Network has grown to include all 53 states and territories (STAT, 2025).

From February 2021 to August 2023, the STAT Reopening K-12 Schools Action Network brought together state education officials, senior public health officials, and COVID-19 task force directors to address the operational challenges faced by STAT members in keeping school communities healthy and open for learning. Since 2023, the STAT Network no longer focuses on school reopening, but its members continue to meet and collaborate on public health challenges, including student mental health, sexual health, violence prevention, and more. Additionally, the seeds planted by STAT have sprouted into a legacy of similar peer-to-peer groups for professionals in the public health and education spaces led by the CDC, the Association for State and Territorial Health Officials (ASTHO), and others.

Competence

Competence, the third dimension of relational trust, reveals itself through knowledge, sound decisions, and reliable follow-through-especially under pressure. Another way to put it is being able to do one's job well. When families trust a school, it is because they believe educators and leaders are not just committed but capable. During the pandemic, that trust extended far beyond academics. Families needed to feel confident that their children would be safe inside school buildings. In many districts, that confidence came to rest on two pivotal roles: school nurses and the district nurse leaders who supported them.

School nurses and district nurse leaders bring a unique blend of clinical expertise and deep understanding of school systems. This positioned them to guide districts through rapidly changing guidance and daily decision-making. School nurses demonstrated competence not just by knowing which mitigation strategies to use, but by understanding how and when to use them and why they worked. They translated public health guidance into action, worked with district leaders to shape policy, solved problems, and helped schools implement mitigation measures. As Dr. Deborah D'Souza-Vazirani of the National Association of School Nurses put it, "School nurses played a pivotal role during the pandemic as the public health experts in schools. They worked with school leaders to educate staff and families and made public health guidance understandable and actionable." Yet in many places, a longstanding shortage of school nurses made this work harder. The pandemic did not create the problem—it exposed it. A 2017 report found that fewer than 40% of U.S. public schools had a full-time nurse (Jean, 2022). Even so, school nurse leaders and their district counterparts across the country stepped up and stretched limited resources to meet overwhelming needs.

Effective leaders demonstrate competence by delegating based on expertise and assuring stakeholders that decisions are made by those with knowledge and experience. In Fulton County, Georgia, for example, Lynne Meadows, the district's longtime director of health services, served on the public health board. This position is not traditionally filled by someone with health expertise, but the Board and the Superintendent of Fulton County Schools recognized the importance of including Meadows, who had cross-sector credibility, built through a combined 30 years of experience in hospital settings, public health, and school nursing. Meadows was a vital bridge between public health and education which enabled Fulton County Schools to mount a rapid and coordinated response. Reflecting on the sheer number and type of partnerships needed during a crisis, Meadows advised, "build these relationships before you need them."

Competence also means knowing when to admit uncertainty. Leaders who acknowledge what they do not know create space for others to do the same. Diana Bruce, a school health consultant in Washington, D.C., who led several national and local communities of practice during the pandemic, emphasized this point: "As a facilitator, I wanted to show my own vulnerability, because it gave others permission to be vulnerable, too. We were all honest about what we didn't know. That's where the learning really happened." This kind of openness does not go unnoticed. Jeremiah Hay, associate commissioner of operations strategy and intelligence at the Massachusetts Department of Transitional Assistance, saw how honesty and humility shaped strong partnerships: "There were so many opportunities for 'gotcha' moments—times when partnerships could have fallen apart. But they didn't. One of the most inspirational things about the pandemic was how people came together and got over their egos."

Competent leaders can say, "I don't know," as an invitation for others to learn with them.

Integrity

Trust is not built on competence alone—it also requires honesty, transparency, and follow-through, which is one way to think about the fourth dimension of relational trust, integrity. Integrity requires being honest and transparent about challenges and trade-offs; taking responsibility for the impact of decisions; and upholding ethical principles that prioritize the well-being of students, staff, and communities—principles such as fairness, accountability, and safety. Across the country, K-12 and public health leaders stood behind tough decisions aimed at protecting the most vulnerable, even when those decisions drew sharp criticism. They navigated public scrutiny, politicized narratives, competing priorities, and personal risk. In Louisville, Kentucky, Dr. Eva Stone, manager of district health for Jefferson County Public Schools (JCPS), faced fierce backlash from parents demanding an early return to in-person learning—well before district health officials believed it was safe. "We have all been threatened with lawsuits," Dr. Stone recalled. "There have been times where we had to have colleagues walk us to our cars because people were so angry about mitigation measures. Nurses needed to have a strong constitution." Despite the intensity of the pushback, JCPS leaders stood firm, reaffirming their commitment to doing what they said they were going to do: keeping student and staff safety at the center of their reopening decisions.

When individuals have a history of demonstrating integrity, trust between them grows. When it came to ensuring indoor air was safe to breathe, for example, Sacramento City Unified School District's director of indoor air quality, Chris Ralston, stressed the importance of having strong vendor relationships for his district of almost 48,000 students across 81 schools. "With supplies like air filters and portable sinks in short supply, we needed to be on the top of vendors' priority lists," he explained. Given the high costs of HVAC upgrades, the urgent timeline imposed by the pandemic, and the administrative hurdles involved in releasing funds, Ralston needed partners who could work immediately and get paid later. Because the district had already built trust with vendors, several were willing to accept those terms—and Sacramento City Schools were able to get what they needed when they needed it most.

▶ PUTTING IT ALL TOGETHER

We have explored each dimension—respect, personal regard, competence, and integrity—individually, though they rarely appear in isolation. In practice, trust is cumulative, reciprocal, and dynamic. The experience of Oregon School District (OSD) in Wisconsin, introduced earlier in the chapter by Superintendent Bergstrom, illustrates how these elements reinforce each other in real time. Bergstrom began thinking about reopening plans the day schools closed in March 2020. She was uncertain what this would look like, but she knew she had partnerships in place to make this happen safely. The district's long-standing relationship with Dr. Jonathan Temte and Shari Barlow with the University of Wisconsin, Madison and the local health department, laid the groundwork for launching a districtwide rapid testing program and reopening schools.

Temte and Barlow were not just experts from the University of Wisconsin. They were neighbors, parents of public-school children, colleagues, and partners who had earned the community's trust long before the pandemic began. Their visible, long-standing presence in the district helped staff and families view them not as distant researchers, but as invested members of the school community. Their work began in 2014 when OSD and the University of Wisconsin partnered on a CDC–sponsored study that explored whether school absences due to respiratory illness could serve as an early warning signal of community-wide outbreaks. The idea was simple: if districts could detect rising respiratory symptoms early, they could act preemptively. They could implementi brief closures, move to a hybrid schedule, or mandate enhanced mitigation strategies while in school (i.e., masking, physical distancing), to prevent further spread, reduce illness, and avoid unnecessary absences (He et al., 2024, 2025). In the study, parent participants reported a child's absence to the district and noted any respiratory-related symptoms, including cough, congestion, and wheezing. The district entered the absence into their systems and shared the reasons for the student's absence with the research team. Within 24 hours, the team conducted a home visit to test the student for respiratory viruses. Families appreciated these home visits. The program offered not just answers, but also incentives: a $50 gift card per family participant, totaling over $165,000 to date in gift cards to local businesses.

When COVID-19 emerged, the groundwork was already in place for the district and university to develop a collaborative response. In 2021–22, the same research team launched a districtwide rapid testing initiative across all seven OSD schools. They trained health office staff, provided testing supplies, and created a seamless results reporting process. Staff welcomed the convenience of on-site testing for students and colleagues, which eliminated the need to travel to outside testing centers. The study team's efforts also generated national insights into the feasibility and acceptability of school-based testing —critical at a time when very little published information (e.g., Vohra et al., 2021) was available.

Temte, Barlow, and their team's work in the district embodies the four dimensions of relational trust. They showed respect by showing up consistently and providing timely, clear information. They demonstrated personal regard through small but meaningful actions as they made house calls to families with an ill child. They showed competence by managing logistics and data with precision, and they acted with integrity by following through on their local commitments. Temte reflected, "Working with this community has been inspiring and enriching. It's been a delight, and we're honored to work with the school district and the community." This is not just a successful local effort—it is evidence that with the right partnerships, school-based testing could be not only feasible but also accepted and even welcomed. The program's success was not accidental. It was the product of partnership built on trust over time.

The story in Oregon underscores that relational trust does not come from any single action or trait. Relational trust is built across time, through the synergistic impact of demonstrating respect, competence, personal regard, and integrity. The Wisconsin team became trusted messengers by embodying these qualities, a critical idea that we return to in Chapter 4. That trust extended to all team members, whose consistent care, responsiveness, and credibility reflected not only on themselves but on the institutions they represented.

Institutional Trust: Reputations and Representatives

When K-12 and public health partners consistently act with competence, follow through on commitments, and put others first, their actions can elevate trust in the institutions they belong to—whether a university, a district, or a local public health department. For example, when parents believe that teachers care about their children's well-being, over time they are more likely to trust not just the individual teacher, but the school as a whole (Tschannen-Moran, 2014). These personal interactions play a critical role in shaping whether communities engage with, believe in, and rely on entire systems, like education or public health.

The same four dimensions that build trust between individuals—respect, personal regard, competence, and integrity—also shape how people come to trust institutions. Institutional trust depends on more than just direct experience—whether with the organization itself or the people who represent it. It also rests on broader perceptions about the institution: an institution's reputation, its track record, and its history with the community (Schoorman et al., 2007). This kind of trust matters when communities are deciding whether to engage with public health agencies, schools, hospitals, or community-based organizations.

The trust between the Oregon School District and the University of Wisconsin research team did not just reflect confidence in a few individuals. Over time, that relational trust began to shape how the school, local businesses, and surrounding community viewed the university—as a capable, ethical, and caring institution.

Trust in institutions is rarely built overnight. It is built over time when people see competence paired with care, and expertise aligned with their values. Dr. Laurel Williams offers a powerful example of how an institution's reputation for competence and care can foster trust, and encourage families to engage not just with individuals, but with the organization as a whole. Williams, medical director with the Texas Child Mental Health

Care Consortium in Houston, Texas, leads a school-linked tele-health program that operates independently but in partnership with schools across the state. She attributes the program's success, in part, to the trust that families place in her department—not just in individual clinicians. "Because people trust my department and we have a good reputation with the community," she explained, "people are open to working with us." When people believe that an entire organization is reliable, competent, and caring, they are more likely to engage, collaborate, and follow guidance. However, when institutions are seen as prioritizing their own agendas over the well-being of those they serve, trust quickly erodes, especially in communities that have been historically harmed by those same institutions.

When people mistrust an institution, especially in communities whose past trust resulted in deep and lasting harm, rebuilding trust is difficult and takes time,. For generations, Indigenous communities across the United States have faced painful breaches of trust by government, health, and education systems, including children being forcefully removed from their home by the government to attend boarding schools. These histories, along with the chronic underfunding of Tribal health services, broken treaties, and dismissals of Tribal sovereignty, have contributed to a deep legacy of mistrust between Indigenous communities and local, state and federal government agencies.

IN BRIEF: NATIVE AMERICAN BOARDING SCHOOLS

In the 19th and 20th centuries, more than 500 government- and church-run boarding schools were established to forcibly assimilate Indigenous children. Many were separated from their families and punished for speaking their Native languages, wearing traditional clothing, or practicing cultural and spiritual customs. The trauma from these efforts to erase Indigenous identity continues to echo today. Some of the elders who endured these schools as children are still alive, carrying with them the weight of those experiences.

(National Native American Boarding School Healing Coalition, 2020)

Rebuilding trust requires more than effective services—it calls for steady, respectful engagement, genuine partnership, and an ongoing commitment to acknowledge and heal the past. Jason Dropik, a member of the Bad River Band of Lake Superior Chippewa and executive director of the National Indian Education Association, encourages organizations entering Tribal communities to build trust through relationships.

> During times of crisis, the most powerful tools organizations can bring are humility, respect, and a commitment to listen. Our communities carry generations of wisdom, strength, and cultural practices that are vital to any healing or recovery effort. I encourage individuals to approach with the mindset of partnership. Take time to understand the local governance, include Tribal leadership in decision-making, and prioritize cultural safety alongside physical health. Trust is not built in urgency. It is earned through relationships. If we honor that, we can truly walk together in solidarity and resilience.

Dropik reminds us that trust is not something that can be demanded, but something that must be earned—patiently, intentionally, and through genuine relationships. To earn trust, a crisis response plan must be built with communities, not forced upon them. When trust has been broken in profound ways, repairing it requires sustained efforts that acknowledge harm, elevate community voices, and build relationships rooted in respect and accountability. Dr. Emily Haroz and her colleagues at the Center for Indigenous Health have been working to do just that. For over 30 years, the Center, based at the Johns Hopkins Bloomberg School of Public Health, has partnered with Indigenous communities to advance health equity through culturally grounded, community-led public health efforts. During the pandemic, Haroz and her team worked with 27 schools serving families across two Tribal Nations in the Southwest. Rather than imposing a testing program on the schools, they developed a testing program that responded to direct requests from the community. "We provided assistance to facilitate testing in schools to support the return to in-person learning. This support was done at the request of schools," she explained. "In this way, we aimed to respect sovereignty and our partners' decisions about what's best for their community." Haroz's team also shared the data from testing so that K-12 leaders could make their own decisions about mitigation measures. "Our role was to provide the data, not to use the data to tell people what to do. That gave us credibility and engendered trust," she said. Sharing data became an act of respect, reinforcing community autonomy and supporting informed, locally driven decisions.

REFLECTIONS FROM THE FIELD: COMMITTING TO A SHARED GOAL

K-12 leaders like Dr. Robert Machak, superintendent of Woodland School District 50, Illinois, decided to work with a number of different partners whose goals aligned with his own— to keep kids healthy and in school.

The most profound takeaway from the pandemic for me was the realization of the vital role our community partners play in keeping our schools open and our people safe. The Lake County Health Department was invaluable in tracking positive cases and identifying close contacts so we could proactively pinpoint and contain potential outbreaks. Partnering with the University of Illinois was even more important: offering its SHIELD PCR testing program[1] at no cost provided the daily assurance that our district community remained healthy and COVID-free. We made testing available to every student and staff member, offering the test weekly; upon a return to in-person learning, we averaged almost 3,000 tests each week. We would not have been able to reopen our schools without them.

When a student, parent, or staff member did test positive, our community partners were there to help in different but equally important ways. For example, we partnered with Warren Township by loading our school buses with groceries from the township food pantry and new coats, hats, and shoes donated by a local community organization to distribute to families that were quarantining or had no other access to these resources. Our district Internet provider offered free or low-cost Internet connectivity to families in our district struggling economically to ensure home connectivity for students in quarantine who were receiving daily academic support from their teachers remotely.

I am a firm believer that adversity does not build character so much as reveal it. Ironically, the challenges associated with reopening our four schools after the pandemic led to so many good people across our community having the opportunity to present the best versions of themselves. With the commitment and support from our community partners, Woodland became a national model for reentry to in-person learning that was thoughtful, intentional, and focused on the physical and social-emotional well-being of every person connected to our school district.

▶ REPAIRING MISTRUST: THE CASE OF THE UNIVERSITY OF ALABAMA AT BIRMINGHAM AND BIRMINGHAM CITY SCHOOLS

To further illustrate how trust in both individuals and institutions is developed and repaired—we share the story of a school of public health in Alabama that partnered with local school districts in Birmingham to offer COVID-19 testing to students and staff. Developing this collaboration required patience and humility because it unfolded in the shadow of a long and painful history of mistrust in public health systems, particularly among Black communities that had been underserved or harmed by these systems in the past.

As the second year of the COVID-19 pandemic began, mitigation efforts in Alabama schools were not uniformly implemented. While the state had initially responded with strong mitigation measures, including mask mandates and physical distancing, many of those mandates ended by the summer of 2021, as vaccines became more widely available. However, vaccination rates in Alabama were low: by June 2021, fewer than 35% of eligible residents had been vaccinated (Holcombe, 2021).

Faced with this reality the Alabama Department of Public Health asked the School of Public Health at the University of Alabama at Birmingham (UAB) to support COVID-19 testing efforts in K-12 schools. Memories of exploitation and neglect, however, made trust hard to come by. Many community members questioned whether the university had the community's best interests at heart. Some believed that UAB's past engagements lacked reciprocity and care. They recalled instances when researchers entered communities to collect data, then left without sharing the implications of the data they collected and without sharing recommendations for how to use the data to address the needs and concerns of the community.

Preexisting mistrust in public health was especially pronounced in Macon County, Alabama, the site of the infamous U.S. Public Health Service Syphilis Study, commonly referred to as the Tuskegee Study (About the USPHS Syphilis Study, 2023). Conducted between 1932 and 1972, the study involved nearly 600 Black men who were misled into believing they were being treated for "bad blood." Most of the participants were low-income sharecroppers, and the incentives the study offered—free medical care, meals, and burial benefits—were a motivating factor to participate, especially in comparison to their daily earnings.

Participants were never asked to give their consent to be in the study or acknowledge the study's risks. When an effective treatment for syphilis, penicillin, became widely available in 1947, the research team deliberately withheld it from participants. Over time, many participants experienced chronic pain, neurological problems, blindness, and heart disease. Several died from this serious but treatable disease, and others unknowingly passed it on to their spouses and children. Their wives contracted the disease, and some children were born with congenital syphilis. The Tuskegee Study is part of a broader and deeply troubling history of medical experimentation on Black Americans—one that began in the colonial era and continues to shape relationships between Black communities and public health institutions today (Washington, 2006).

Although the Tuskegee Study ended in 1972, it continues to shape how many families and communities of color, especially those directly impacted, view public health institutions. For many, trust has not been easily rebuilt (Alsan et al., 2020). During the pandemic, inaccurate health information about testing and vaccines circulated, fueling confusion and deepening longstanding mistrust in public health. Some people believed they could not get the virus because of their blood type or skin color; others dismissed it as "just the flu" (Planas, 2021). Some thought the virus was a political hoax (Reuters Staff, 2020). Frequent changes to guidance on masking, vaccination, and quarantine added to the uncertainty, making it even harder for public health officials to earn trust and keep communities informed.

K-12 and public health leaders, researchers, scientists, and practitioners in Birmingham were not just professionals—they were also members of the community. Because they lived and worked in the same neighborhoods as the families they served, they were especially attuned to the mistrust many families felt toward UAB, public health institutions more broadly, and recommendations around testing and vaccination. To begin rebuilding trust and increase the number of students and staff being tested on a regular basis public health leaders had to first acknowledge it had been broken and then take visible, sustained steps to repair it. Birmingham City Schools and UAB initiated a variety of activities to build trust in public health recommendations These initiatives included: 1) hosting listening sessions that featured video conversations with descendants of the Tuskegee Study participants; 2) employing community members as school liaisons to explain and support testing; and 3) offering a financial incentive for students and districts to increase participation in school-based testing.

Listening to Tuskegee Descendants

Birmingham City Schools in Alabama is a metropolitan district that serves 21,000 students, 90% of whom identify as Black or African American. As he urged his school community to participate in COVID-19 testing and get vaccinated, Dr. Mark Sullivan, a Black leader serving a predominantly Black community, faced the difficult task of asking families to place their trust in institutions like UAB and public health agencies—entities that, for many, were still associated with the historic betrayal of their grandparents and great-grandparents. In the winter of 2020–2021, as vaccines became more widely available and eligibility expanded, nearly two-thirds of parents in the district reported that they did not plan to get vaccinated themselves—or to have their children vaccinated. Several parents shared that they wanted to see how others responded to the vaccine before making a decision for their own families. Others voiced a deeper concern—that they might be part of an experiment, once again. Sullivan acknowledged these fears, noting that for many, mistrust stemmed not from inaccurate health information, but from real, lived experiences and a long history of being overlooked, under-served, and harmed by the very systems now asking for their trust.

With support from UAB, the district launched a large-scale testing program and set up multiple pop-up clinics, but only a small number of students participated. To increase participation, Sullivan emphasized to families that testing played a critical role in identifying asymptomatic individuals, those who could unknowingly spread the virus, and in preventing potentially serious illness or death. But as superintendent and someone deeply familiar with his school community, he knew that information about the benefits of testing or vaccination alone would not be enough to address mistrust and hesitancy. Sullivan understood that rebuilding trust meant restoring confidence not only in the field itself, but also in the people who represented it and the public health institutions that carried its work forward

Sullivan and his fellow district administrators believed that rebuilding trust had to begin with transparency about health-related decision-making and empathy towards families' fears and lived experiences. They needed to show their genuine willingness to listen to families' questions and hear their concerns, instead of downplaying or judging their uncertainty. As one step toward that, the district hosted listening sessions and screened the U.S. Ad Council's *COVID Conversations*—a video series featuring descendants of Tuskegee Study participants who spoke candidly about why they chose to get tested or vaccinated for COVID-19. Afterward, district leaders facilitated open conversations with families to explore how both historical and present-day injustices have shaped the community's lack of trust in public health. These conversations invited the school community to name what had happened, acknowledge the harm, and reflect on how those experiences continue to shape health-related beliefs and behaviors today. By connecting current fears, frustrations, and anger to long-standing patterns of exclusion, to present day concerns and hesitation, the district helped stakeholders build a shared understanding of where mistrust stems from—and what it might take to begin rebuilding it.

For Sullivan and his team, rebuilding trust in public health was not a one-time event—it was an ongoing strategic effort which also included sharing updates through social media, local radio, and even through door to door knocking and one-on-one conversations. Over time, that effort made a difference. More students and families chose to participate in the testing program and get vaccinated because they felt informed, respected, and heard. The district's work did not go unnoticed. In recognition of their commitment to culturally responsive, community-directed engagement, Birmingham City Schools was awarded a Golden Achievement Award from the National School Public Relations Association (NSPRA) (Puryear, 2022), which recognizes a district's outstanding work in communication and community partnership. The honor reflected not only what the district accomplished, but how they did it—by listening first, building trust, and showing that public health could be a partner, not just a presence or imposition, in the lives of families they serve.

At its core, the district's effort was about more than increasing participation in testing or vaccination—it was about restoring trust in a system that, for many families, had long felt distant or even harmful. Institutional trust is shaped not only by an organization's actions, but also by how those actions are perceived—through the lens of history, lived experience, and reputation. In Alabama, and particularly among families in Birmingham City Schools, trust in the broader public health system was fractured. But relational trust—trust in the people who represent that system—opened the door to something deeper. As a trusted leader within the school community, Sullivan stood alongside families and spoke on behalf of the institution of public health with empathy and honesty. In doing so, he helped reframe what public health could be: not a distant authority, but a responsive and trustworthy partner.

School Liaisons: Building Trust in the Community Through the Community

Two miles northwest of Birmingham City Schools sits the University of Alabama at Birmingham (UAB). Though close in distance, the two institutions, like many urban universities and public-school systems, often operate in separate worlds. At UAB, the median family income for students is over $80,000; in Birmingham City Schools, it hovers just above $40,000, with nearly 1,700 students experiencing some form of homelessness. As the fall 2021 semester began, those differences gave way to a shared uncertainty about what was coming. Just as students, staff, and families were settling back into in-person learning, the Delta variant swept through the South.

Unlike earlier phases of the pandemic when most districts closed, this time, districts stayed open. However, they struggled to keep up with evolving risks and limited resources, often implementing short-term, reactive closures in response to school-based outbreaks. To support districts, the Alabama Department of Public Health enlisted UAB's School of Public Health to lead voluntary COVID-19 testing and infection prevention efforts for K-12 students and staff statewide. The initiative was part of a national strategy coordinated by the CDC and funded by the American Rescue Plan Act of 2021, through which the U.S. Department of Health and Human Services allocated $10 billion to support testing in K-12 schools.

To increase participation in testing, UAB added a new role to the school-based testing team: the school liaison. Liaisons were trusted community members, often retired teachers, school nurses, bus drivers, or parents, who supported the day-to-day logistics of testing. They helped in practical, hands-on ways: escorting students from class to the testing room or covering a teacher's class so that teacher could get tested. According to Dr. Angela Sullivan, program director, these small but essential tasks made a big difference for school building staff, students, and families. School liaisons listened carefully to concerns and responded without judgment. They understood the testing program and partnered with the testing team to explain the process in reassuring, accessible ways. They reassured young students, "You'll feel a little tickle, but it won't tickle your brain," and offered to hold their hands. Because liaisons came from the same communities as the students and families they served, they were often familiar and friendly and well positioned to build trust.

School liaisons effectiveness went beyond familiarity. At a moment when many students were still recovering from social disconnection and disrupted routines, liaisons offered calm, consistency, and care. They were trusted adults who showed up week after week, ready to listen, explain, and ease anxiety. That steady presence helped normalize testing and strengthen the connective tissue in school communities at a time when togetherness and a sense of belonging was vital. Their ongoing presence gave students something every school community needs: trusted adults who consistently show up. The relationships that liaisons built with students and staff left a lasting impression, so much so that many continued working in schools even after the testing program ended. As trust grew, more families enrolled their children in school-based testing programs, and testing rates steadily increased.

The school liaisons' work in Alabama was shaped by the four dimensions of relational trust. First, they listened with respect to students, families, and staff without judgment or defensiveness. Second, they showed genuine personal regard, asking how students were doing, remembering names, and checking in again the next week. Third, they were compentent. Liaisons were well trained, understood the testing process, and could answer questions or connect families to someone who could. And finally, they acted with integrity—showing up not once, but consistently, with dedication and determination.

Offering Meaningful Incentives to Test

In the summer of 2022, the nation reached a grave milestone: more than one million Americans had died from COVID-19. Just months earlier, the Omicron variant had driven a sharp surge in hospitalizations and deaths, with weekly numbers in January and February nearing the highest levels of the entire pandemic. Widespread testing and vaccination had already proven effective in preventing illness and death by identifying asymptomatic individuals who were unknowingly spreading the virus. This "silent spread" posed a particular threat to elders in multigenerational households and to unvaccinated individuals. However, in Alabama, student participation in school-based testing remained low, and as of August 2022, only 64% of Alabamans had even had one dose of the COVID-19 vaccine (USA Facts, 2025).

Faced with rising case numbers and low participation, the UAB testing team knew that doing more of the same would not be enough—so they paused, reached out, and asked school communities directly: *What would make this work for you?* The answer was clear: *resources for our schools and districts.* This response became the starting point for an innovative testing strategy, one based on the everyday needs of school communities. Beginning in fall 2022, districts would receive $40,000 if at least one school building offered testing; schools would receive $15,000 for holding at least one testing event; and each student would receive a $15 gift card every week that they tested. After the incentive program was launched, student testing rates across the state increased significantly. In the year prior to the incentive component, 223 schools participated in UAB's testing program, which administered over 141,000 tests statewide (Tryens-Fernandes, 2022). The following year, 814 schools enrolled in the program, a 73% increase, and over 900,000 tests, an 84% increase, were administered across Alabama (White, 2023).

In addition to the financial benefit, the incentive program had a meaningful impact for several reasons. It helped students think critically about the power of collective action and gave them a deeper understanding of what it means to participate in a public health effort. Superintendent Sullivan shared that "several of the community members mentioned that the incentive piece got a lot of the students wondering how this might translate into their future careers in healthcare or public health." Those conversations revealed something powerful: the incentives were not just motivating participation; they were prompting students to think about their own futures. While a gift card alone cannot build trust, thoughtfully designed incentives that demonstrate care and responsiveness can open the door.

The program's success, reflected in higher testing rates, was made possible by the growing trust between families, students, and public health leaders. UAB and its partners demonstrated that trust in four essential ways. First, they showed respect by listening closely to school communities and responding directly to what they heard. Second, they demonstrated personal regard by offering meaningful support, recognizing not just the seriousness of the moment, but the value of each individual's well-being. Third, they showed competence by placing well-trained liaisons and community partners on-site, ready to answer questions and guide implementation. And fourth, they showed integrity and follow through. Schools and districts received the support they were promised, and students who tested regularly received weekly gift cards. By centering trust in both the design and the delivery of the program, the UAB team and its partners didn't just increase participation in testing—they helped rebuild confidence in public health and strengthened the relationships that hold school communities together.

▶ TRUST CAN BE REBUILT: LESSONS FROM ALABAMA

Through strong expressions of relational trust, UAB and Birmingham City Schools helped rebuild community confidence in a public health institution and public health recommendations. Their collaboration illustrated different ways to build trust with communities, helping families see public health institutions as aligned with their need to feel safe, healthy, respected and heard. Across Alabama, public health officials, K-12 administrators, and university partners worked side by side with families and educators to bring students back into classrooms as quickly and safely as possible. Trusted messengers, including community-based school liaisons and large-scale public campaigns, helped

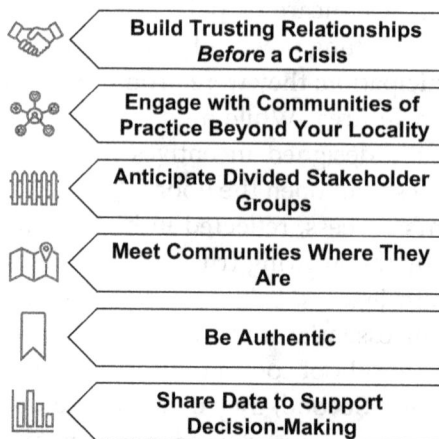

	Build Trusting Relationships *Before* a Crisis
	Engage with Communities of Practice Beyond Your Locality
	Anticipate Divided Stakeholder Groups
	Meet Communities Where They Are
	Be Authentic
	Share Data to Support Decision-Making

Figure 2.2 Considerations for Building and Maintaining Trust.

communicate the benefits of testing and vaccination. Financial incentives for both schools and families encouraged participation, and the visible success of in-person learning with minimal COVID-19 transmission reinforced the community's belief in safety plans. Over time, trust grew, not only between families and public health leaders, but across organizations. School liaisons, community members, UAB, and state agencies forged relationships by working together to repair trust and achieve the common goal of keeping kids safe and in school.

▶ CONSIDERATIONS FOR BUILDING AND MAINTAINING TRUSTING PARTNERSHIPS

Strong partnerships made reopening districts during the pandemic possible. Building on those lessons, we now outline specific actions leaders can take to establish and sustain trust at both the relational and institutional levels. While cultivating relational trust is a vital starting point, leaders must also invest in strengthening trust in institutions—this trust endures beyond individual relationships, leadership transitions, or temporary incentives. By doing so, leaders can create resilient systems that invest in cultivating the types of partnerships and collaborations that keep students safe, supported, and learning—during crises and beyond.

Build Trusting Relationships Before a Crisis

The work of reopening schools highlights the importance of partnering with a wide range of organizations—both traditional and nontraditional. From university researchers and public health agencies to for-profit manufacturers of personal protective equipment, cleaning supplies, test kits, and vaccines, districts need to identify reliable partners to act quickly and effectively.

Strong relationships with trusted partners do not happen overnight—they need to be established and nurtured well before a crisis. To begin, leaders can identify key organizations in their communities and being to develop relationships. See Appendix C for resources to help identify and develop new partnerships and to strengthen existing partnerships.

Engage with Communities of Practice Beyond Your Locality

A trusted community of practice (COP, Wenger, 1998) offers leaders another type of partner and support during crisis, as they come together with others who share their role to address the same critical issue. When leaders are navigating uncharted territory, finding peers in similar organizations can offer significant sources of support. If you are the superintendent of your school district, you may be the only superintendent within your geographic area. COPs provide space for collegiality, empathy, and collective problem solving. Strong COPs create a safe space for leaders who may be unaccustomed to not knowing the correct decision to make and who need a welcoming, non-judgmental space to ask questions and seek advice. COPs keep leaders connected and learning, instead of isolated.

COPs can also serve as effective platforms to bring in subject matter experts who can provide technical and tactical guidance specific to the nature of the crisis. At the same time, experts benefit from listening to practitioners' conversations, learning directly from the experiences of those on the ground. They can engage participants in discussions about the feasibility and acceptability of different approaches. Sometimes COPs can be well-funded initiatives supported by external organizations; other times, they can be informal groups of leaders with a shared concern. Either way, connecting with individuals who share similar responsibilities and challenges can lead to collective problem solving, anticipatory planning (as one district or state discusses an issue or event that will soon affect others), and validation – as as leaders recognize that their struggles are shared and their efforts are valued.

Anticipate Divided Stakeholder Groups

Building trust during a crisis is difficult and often deeply personal. Leaders can find themselves in the middle of a national debate playing out at the local level as constituents argue passionately on different sides of the issue. In this type of divided landscape, meetings can quickly unravel. Navigating disagreement while maintaining trust is an essential and difficult leadership skill. Anticipating that divisions will occur positions leaders to develop initiatives that are responsive to community concerns. Empathy and a deep respect for people's autonomy and lived experiences can support leaders as they work with divided groups. Showing respect for individuals with opposing viewpoints and ensuring that everyone has a chance to share their concerns can keep conversations constructive. Leaders can demonstrate positive intent—trusting that colleagues and partners are here to help, even if they see things differently—and ask that individuals also work to assume good intent. Framing disagreements around ideas and solutions rather than people and allowing individuals to speak without interruption can also foster constructive dialogue across difference.

These practices will not erase conflict, but they create the conditions for it to be aired productively—and for trust to deepen, even in difficult conversations. When the stakes are high and the environment turns hostile, leaders are most successful when they understand their communities and can anticipate likely issues that will cause division.

Meet Communities Where They Are

Meeting communities where they are means learning about community members' priorities and concerns, instead of assuming communities share priorities and concerns. This can literally mean meeting people where they are, geographically, holding events in different locations across a district or community or visiting students' houses for check-ins and conversation. It can also include hosting events to elicit community feedback and discussion.

This can also mean meeting communities where they are in terms of their concerns and needs. For example, if a community is hesitant about vaccination, a district might choose to slow down its vaccination campaign and instead focus on education about the vaccine and offer town halls with medical experts to discuss concerns. Focusing on the newest technology or educational platform is not useful for a district if most families do not have devices or internet access at home. Learning from the community means that leaders may need to change their course of action.

Be Authentic

Being authentic means being yourself and being willing to admit what you do not know. This kind of honesty can go a long way, though it often can feel scary. Leaders who acknowledge their own uncertainties create space for others to share their uncertainty too. Often, this vulnerability does not weaken trust, but instead invites others to be vulnerable, which can strengthen trust. In contrast, pretending to have all the answers causes distance when everyone knows that many answers are still unknown.

Share Data to Support Decision-Making

Trust often hinges on transparency. One of the most effective ways leaders can create trust is by sharing data early, often, and accessibly. Public-facing dashboards that visualize real-time data, trends, and potential impacts help communities to understand why decisions are being made, and help individuals make their own decisions. By sharing timely, reliable, and actionable information, institutions that collect data show what it means to treat families, educators, and community members as full participants in the work of keeping communities safe. Making data visible can help calm fears, answer questions, and create a shared understanding of what is happening—and what needs to happen next. Data transparency, especially in places without formal mandates to share data gives families and educators a sense of agency.

▶ PUTTING TRUST TO WORK: ADDRESSING INEQUITY AS A THREAT TO THE PUBLIC'S HEALTH

Throughout the pandemic, trust between public health and K-12 leaders made it possible for districts to act quickly and bring students safely back into classrooms. However, in many communities, the absence of trust between marginalized communities and institutions stymied reopening efforts Building trust is not enough for a strong response if it overlooks the inequities that have long undermined it. To keep all children safe, leaders must plan with these inequities in mind, ensuring that crisis responses do not repeat or deepen past harms. While trust lays the groundwork for strong partnerships, addressing inequities ensures those partnerships truly serve every child. In the next chapter, we turn to equity and explore how centering it can strengthen K–12 and public health partnerships and help keep students safe and in school during public health crises.

▶ NOTE

1 SHIELD Illinois is discussed in greater depth in Chapter 3.

References

About the USPHS Syphilis Study. (2023). Tuskegee University. Retrieved from https://www.tuskegee.edu/about-us/centers-of-excellence/bioethics-center/about-the-usphs-syphilis-study

Alsan, M., Wanamaker, M., & Hardeman, R. R. (2020). The Tuskegee study of untreated syphilis: A case study in peripheral trauma with implications for health professionals. *Journal of General Internal Medicine, 35*, 322–325.

Bryk, A. S., & Schneider, B. (2003). Trust in schools: A core resource for school reform. *Educational Leadership, 60*(6), 40–45.

Gillon, R. (2003). Ethics needs principles: Four can encompass the rest—and respect for autonomy should be "first among equals". *Journal of Medical Ethics, 29*(5), 307–312.

Hallam, P. R., & Hausman, C. (2009). Principal and teachers relations: Trust at the core of school improvement. In *International handbook of research on teachers and teaching* (pp. 403–416). Boston, MA: Springer US.

He, C., Goss, M., Norton, D., Chen, G., Uzicanin, A., & Temte, J. (2025). Effects of K-12 school district non-pharmaceutical interventions on community-level prevalence of acute respiratory infection during the COVID-19 pandemic. *Authorea.* https://doi.org/10.22541/au.174187454.44705515/v1

He, C., Norton, D., Temte, J. L., Barlow, S., Goss, M., Temte, E., Bell, C., Chen, G., & Uzicanin, A. (2024). Effect of planned school breaks on student absenteeism due to influenza-like illness in school aged children: Oregon School District, Wisconsin September 2014–June 2019. *Influenza and Other Respiratory Viruses*, *18*(1), e13244.

Holcombe, M. (2021). The Delta variant will cause 'very dense outbreaks' in these five states, expert says. *CNN Health*. Retrieved from https://www.cnn.com/2021/06/28/health/us-coronavirus-monday/index.html

Jean, J. Y. (2022). Why school nurses are leaving the career. *Nurse Journal*. Retrieved from https://nursejournal.org/articles/why-school-nurses-are-leaving/

Louis, K. S. (2007). Trust and improvement in schools. *Journal of Educational Change*, *8*(1), 1–24.

National Native American Boarding School Healing Coalition (2020). Retrieved from https://boardingschoolhealing.org/

Pandi-Perumal, S. R., Vaccarino, S. R., Chattu, V. K., Zaki, N. F., BaHammam, A. S., Manzar, D., ... & Kennedy, S. H. (2021). 'Distant socializing,' not 'social distancing' as a public health strategy for COVID-19. *Pathogens and Global Health*, *115*(6), 357–364.

Planas, A. (2021). 'It's too late': Alabama doctor shares final moments of Covid patients, urges vaccination. *NBC News*. Retrieved from https://www.nbcnews.com/news/us-news/it-s-too-late-alabama-doctor-shares-final-moments-covid-n1274659

Puryear, C. (2022). BREAKING: Birmingham City Schools wins national award for COVID-19 campaign. *Bham Now*. Retrieved from https://bhamnow.com/2022/06/23/birmingham-city-schools-covid-19-campaign/

Puyallup Tribe of Indians. (n.d.). spuyaləpabš: syəcəb ʔə tiiɬ ʔiišədčəɬ (Puyallup Tribe: The Story of Our People). Retrieved from https://puyallup-tribe.com/ourtribe/

Reuters Staff. (2020). Fact check: Alabama nurse did not die after receiving the COVID-19 vaccine. Retrieved from https://www.reuters.com/article/world/fact-check-alabama-nurse-did-not-die-after-receiving-the-covid-19-vaccine-idUSKBN28S2FA/

Schoorman, F. D., Mayer, R. C., & Davis, J. H. (2007). An integrative model of organizational trust: Past, present, and future. *Academy of Management Review*, *32*(2), 344–354.

STAT. (2025). The Rockefeller foundation. Retrieved from https://www.rockefellerfoundation.org/covid-19-response/stat/

Tryens-Fernandes, S. (2022). UAB extends free child COVID testing, works with schools to attract more students. AL. Com. Retrieved from https://www.al.com/news/2022/09/uab-extends-free-child-covid-testing-works-with-schools-to-attract-more-students.html

Tschannen-Moran, M. (2014). The interconnectivity of trust in schools. In Forsyth, P. B., Van Houtte, M., & Van Maele, D. (Eds.). *Trust and School Life: The Role of Trust for Learning, Teaching, Leading, and Bridging.* (57–81), Netherlands: Springer.

USA Facts. (2025). US coronavirus vaccine tracker. Retrieved from https://usafacts.org/visualizations/covid-vaccine-tracker-states/

Vohra, D., Rowan, P., Hotchkiss, J., Lim, K., Lansdale, A., & O'Neil, S. (2021). Implementing COVID-19 routine testing in K-12 schools: Lessons and recommendations from pilot sites. *Mathematica.* https://files.eric.ed.gov/fulltext/ED614674.pdf

Washington, H. A. (2006). *Medical apartheid: The dark history of medical experimentation on Black Americans from colonial times to the present.* Doubleday Books.

Wenger, E. (1998). Communities of practice: Learning as a social system. *Systems Thinker, 9*(5), 2–3.

White, M. (2023). COVID-19 Testing and Prevention in Alabama's K-12 Schools program wraps up with 925,000 tests, 814 schools enrolled and more than 24,000 student participants. *UAB News.* Retrieved from https://www.uab.edu/news/health/item/13795-alabama-s-covid-19-k-12-testing-and-prevention-program-wraps-up-with-925-000-tests-814-schools-enrolled-and-more-than-24-000-student-participants#:~:text=Health%20%26%20Medicine-,COVID%2D19%20Testing%20and%20Prevention%20in%20Alabama's%20K%2D12%20Schools,more%20than%2024%2C000%20student%20participants

Advancing Equity

Planning from the Margins

In the summer of 2021, we approached the return to school with the idea of designing from the margins and how to make sure that we reached all our families. We worked with an outside organization to get input from families across Massachusetts, and to oversample families from marginalized populations. We used information from those listening sessions to design the program for our relaunch and help us to communicate using parent-friendly language. Planning from the margins really set us up for the trajectory of the next school year.

> Dr. Russell Johnston, (former) Acting Commissioner,
> Massachusetts Department of Elementary
> and Secondary Education

As K-12 districts and states developed plans to reopen schools, they needed to make sure that these plans would work for all families and students. To do so, they worked with public health organizations, community partners, researchers and the private sector to plan from the margins—to think about those who were on the outside edge of their communities and thus less able to access health services and up-to-date information about the pandemic. For Johnston, planning from the margins meant reaching out to families to learn more about what they needed to ensure a safe and feasible return to in-person learning after more than a year out of school. Instead of thinking about a

DOI: 10.4324/9781003608844-3

"typical" student or family, planning from the margins requires leaders to consider the needs of those who are the least likely to be given access to tangible resources, information, and decision-making opportunities.

In this chapter, we argue that planning from the margins is a useful way to think about equity. K-12 and public health leaders can use this approach to help their organizations and communities prepare for, respond to, and recover from public health crises. When partners share a clear definition of equity, they can develop fair, responsive programs, policies, and practices that promote health, education, and wellness for all.

We begin this chapter by defining what it means to plan from the margins. Next, we introduce two key strategies for planning from the margins: first, prioritizing limited resources to serve those with the greatest need; and second, tailoring the level and type of support to ensure that resources are available, accessible, and useful to diverse stakeholder groups. We then examine the case of Jefferson County Public Schools in Louisville, Kentucky, where district and public health leaders partnered to implement a testing program amid historical racial inequities, significant linguistic diversity, and a state-level COVID-19 response with limited mandated mitigation. This case illustrates a district's commitment to reaching students on the margins, particularly students of color and those whose families speak other languages in addition to English, and how this commitment helped them design a broad-reaching testing program, accessible to district families and the broader community. We conclude by outlining key steps that K-12 and public health partners can take to create equitable processes that center and support students and families on the margins—and, in doing so, better serve all families.

▶ HOW TO CENTER EQUITY IN A CRISIS

When schools moved to remote learning in the fall of 2020, and later to in-person or hybrid models, longstanding inequities in access to education, technology, and support, - often hidden from view - became impossible to ignore. During the pandemic, students with disabilities, students from low-income families, English language learners, undocumented students, transient students, and those living in rural areas continued to face greater barriers to learning and experienced lower levels of academic success (Crow, 2022). These students lacked access to many critical resources and supports, including personal protective equipment (PPE) like face masks, hand sanitizer, and soap; tools for remote or hybrid learning, such as internet access, reliable bandwidth, laptops, tablets, and quiet spaces; teachers with experience or training in virtual instruction; and social supports, including peers and trusted school personnel.

For K-12 and public health partnerships to promote the health and academic success of all students, they must start by attending to students who face these barriers. In practice, planning from the margins means considering the needs of students who have more barriers or who have experienced less success from the outset. Planning with those at the margins in mind tends to strengthen policies overall, unlike general plans that require multiple "add-ons" to patch gaps after the fact.

Andrea Cahn, senior vice president of Unified Champion Schools at Special Olympics, has spent over 35 years advancing inclusion for students with intellectual and developmental disabilities (ID/DD). During the pandemic, one of the greatest challenges was ensuring these students, already at risk for social isolation and exclusion, were not overlooked or left behind as schools made decisions about reopening. However, Cahn reflected that

> return-to-school policies were done from a general education mindset first and then districts developed plans to deal with the special education population afterward. What we learned is that all decisions about our schools have to take all students into account. The student body is a body and has to be treated as a whole body.

When K-12 and public health partners fail to plan from the margins, existing health and academic disparities tend to deepen. For students with ID/DD, who were more likely to die from COVID-19 infections (Turk et al., 2020), returning to school required stricter mitigation measures than the general population. Their needs were often not met by return-to-school plans that accounted for the needs of *most* students. As a result of generic policies, many parents of students with ID/DD chose to keep their children home, sacrificing instructional time and peer connections, because their students' health needs had not been adequately considered. However, when leaders begin by addressing the needs of the most vulnerable, the result is a responsive system that supports the entire student body.

REFLECTIONS FROM THE FIELD: PARTNERING TO HELP STUDENTS WITH DISABILITIES SUCCEED

John Eisenberg, executive director with the National Association of State Directors of Special Education, found that when partners centered the needs of students with disabilities, continuous learning was a very real possibility.

> The COVID-19 pandemic underscored the vital need for consistent and structured communication between special education leaders and public health authorities. Approximately 14% of K-12 students have disabilities requiring specialized instruction, with many also needing medical interventions and ongoing health support throughout their education. The crisis highlighted the value of robust collaboration and regular dialogue with public health partners. Special education stakeholders relied extensively on guidance and recommendations from public health agencies, enabling many students to sustain their educational progress despite significant disruptions to in-person learning. This partnership proved instrumental in navigating the challenges and ensuring continuity of learning for students with disabilities.

K–12 leaders who have applied Universal Design for Learning (UDL) principles, developed by the Center for Applied Special Technology in the late 1990s, are likely familiar with this approach. UDL helps teachers attend to the variability in how students learn and encourages them to design lessons and assignments that are accessible to all students. When a curriculum is universally designed, students have options to engage in learning in ways that are most effective and meaningful for them (Rose et al., 2002). This might mean, for example, letting students choose from a hands-on activity, an individual pencil and paper exercise, or a group discussion. Creating this type of learning environment demonstrates respect for the different ways that students learn and a commitment to the dignity and agency of learners. Considering the needs of students at the margins should be extended to planning for crises as well. This work, as highlighted by Johnston in the opening of this chapter, begins with understanding what students on the margins need to feel supported and continue learning during a crisis.

To do this, a district might collaborate with a university or community-based partner to design a simple survey or interview protocol design a simple survey or interview protocol that helps district leaders learn more about their communities. This process can reveal the specific barriers to learning faced by students on the margins, and, in the ideal world, guide a plan that ensures uninterrupted learning and support. A plan designed around the margins not only prevents disruption for the most vulnerable but also ensures that every student has the support to keep learning.

However, to plan from the margins and lead with equity, a common language and shared definitions are needed, especially around what terms like *access* and *equity* mean. They also need a shared understanding of the problem. For instance, if the long-term goal is to improve regular attendance because of high absenteeism rates, the district first needs to understand why students are absent. A district might develop a simple tracking system and establish a FERPA- and HIPAA-compliant data-sharing agreement with local medical centers. After gathering data from this system, they would reach out to families of students who are regularly absent. Partners can tailor their responses: if illness is the main reason for absences, districts might expand access to testing or vaccination; if transportation is a barrier, districts might adjust bus routes or change start times; if mental health is a concern, leaders could increase access to school counselors and explore telehealth options.

IN BRIEF: WHAT ARE FERPA AND HIPAA, AND WHY DO THEY MATTER IN SCHOOLS?

FERPA (Family Educational Rights and Privacy Act) is a federal law that protects the privacy of students' education records—including attendance, grades, and health-related information maintained by schools. In K-12 settings, it is typically the responsibility of the school district to ensure FERPA compliance, often managed by district data teams, administrators, and legal counsel.

HIPAA (Health Insurance Portability and Accountability Act) protects the confidentiality of individuals' personal health information when it is handled by healthcare providers. In most cases, HIPAA applies to healthcare entities, not to schools—but when districts partner with public health or other outside agencies, HIPAA–compliant systems may be necessary for secure data exchange.

Why It Matters: During a public health crisis, districts may need to share or receive sensitive health data to coordinate services like testing, vaccination, or mental health support. Ensuring compliance with FERPA and HIPAA protects student privacy, builds trust with families, and helps partnerships operate legally.

To create meaningful, lasting change for underserved and overlooked students, especially during times of crisis, K–12 and public health leaders can work with communities, organizations, and people that shape the daily experiences of these students. This approach acknowledges that multiple interrelated factors influence how students learn and grow. These factors operate at different levels of a student's social environment: family and friends (individual), school, neighborhood, and district (organizational), and broader policy systems (community). Thinking about equity across levels helps leaders to understand that people are shaped by the environments around them (Bronfenbrenner, 1977). This approach also encourages leaders to leverage each level to build stronger, synergistic supports for every child. In the following sections, we share examples of what it means to plan from the margins at each of these levels.

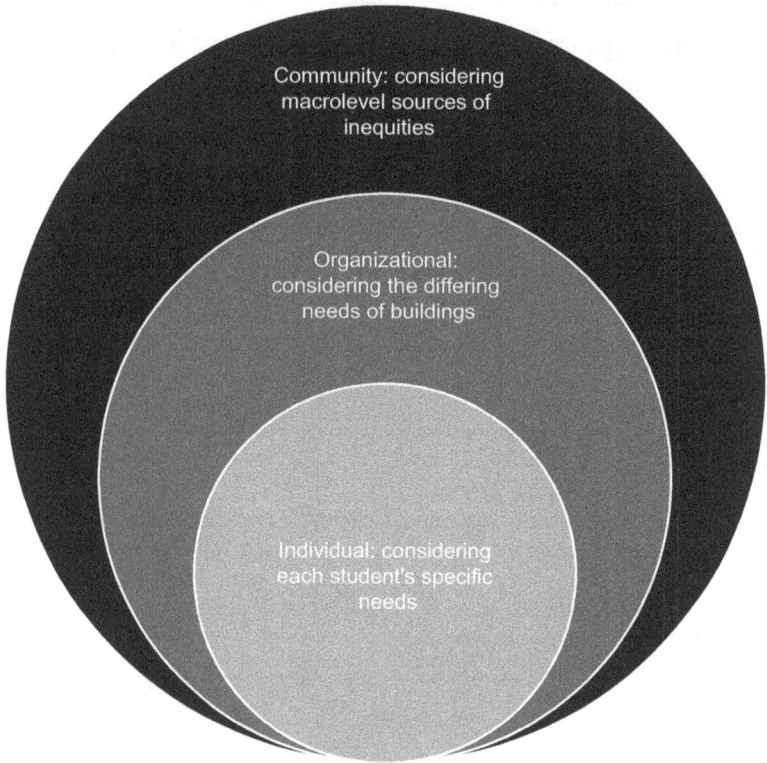

Figure 3.1 Levels of Equity in K-12 and Public Health Work.

Planning from the Margins at the Individual Level

Planning from the margins at the individual level means considering the specific needs, strengths, and circumstances of each student and family. Addressing equity at this level requires not only understanding concerns and needs, such as continued access to school meals during closures, but also recognizing and drawing on the strengths that families bring.

During the pandemic, many districts gathered this kind of information using short online or paper surveys. Multiple-choice surveys offer a relatively quick way to gather insights from a broad group of stakeholders. (See Appendix E for tips on creating your own community survey.) Follow-up interviews and focus groups can then help clarify and expand on patterns seen in the survey data. For example, a survey might show how many families lack access to high-speed internet. Focus groups or interviews can help identify what type of access would be most useful, such as mobile hotspot devices, hotspot access via smart-phones, or internet provided at a central community location.

REFLECTIONS FROM THE FIELD: ENGAGING THE COMMUNITY

Brittany Choate, director of programs for SalivaDirect at Yale University's School of Public Health, emphasized that successful public health efforts, especially those aimed at traditionally underserved communities, must begin with genuine community engagement.

> Local public health perspectives and community-driven solutions must be incorporated into the program design to achieve meaning-ful, long-lasting results. This is especially true when seeking to sup-port traditionally underserved communities. Taking time to build relationships with established, trusted community partners will allow you to leverage their connections and glean insights from their on-the-ground knowledge, such as existing resources or paral-lel programs and how to develop culturally informed strategies.
> Embracing an iterative engagement model with partners and community members is key—listen, ask for input, revise, and repeat these steps throughout the program's life. This will uncover evolv-ing public health challenges and opportunities, which can be used to inform next steps and ensure the program offers value. All of this, in turn, will improve resource allocation and efficiency of your pro-gram, but more importantly, will increase trust, buy-in, and partici-pation from your community.

Meeting the needs of individual students and families during a public health crisis often calls for creativity, compassion, and adaptability. For example, rather than requiring medically frag-ile students who could not wear masks to stay home, a district in Oregon used clear shower curtains to create physical dividers between students, allowing them to remain in the classroom while reducing the risk for transmission. Across the country in New Jersey's North Brunswick Township Schools, Mary Ellen Engel, then the district's nursing supervisor, and her team designed a sensory-friendly COVID-19 testing and vaccination clinic. Engel created this clinic in response to listening to and learning from families with children who received special education services. Families shared that clinical settings, medical procedures, and unfamiliar environments often triggered anxiety or fear in their children, leading to canceled appointments and delays in care. To ensure these students had equitable access to school-based health services, Engel collaborated with parents and special education teachers to design a space that was less stimulating and more comforting. The space minimized bright lighting, loud noises, and visible medical equipment. Students bypassed traditional clinical areas, met with familiar teachers and staff, and received care in a quiet room. Comforts included sensory tools like fidget items and calming visuals—all designed to reduce stress and support participation. Without those thoughtful adaptations, some families may have continued delaying or avoiding testing and vaccination altogether.

Unfortunately, even the most creative strategies, robust data systems, and deep commitment to equity could not replace the basics, including proper PPE and trained personnel. Without these in place, some medically vulnerable students were unable to return to in-person learning for more than two years. Supporting these students required customized virtual learning schedules to ensure they had access to experienced and certified teachers. To meet each student's individual needs, paraprofessionals, speech-language pathologists, audiologists, and occupational therapists began connecting with families through video conferences and, when possible, home visits.

An unexpected benefit of the shift to virtual learning was that it gave many parents a window into the broad scope and depth of services their children received at school. Dr. L. Penny Rosenblum, research professor emerita at the University of Arizona, referred to this as a silver lining:

> families got a better understanding of professionals, and parents who might not have known how best to support their child with completing tasks at home, like making their own snacks, now were more empowered to do so because they could follow the steps the teachers explained on [the video conference].

Rosenblum highlighted how virtual learning gave families insight into how their children learned and how to support them at home. At the same time, educators and specialists also gained a deeper understanding of students' home learning environments. Eric Masten, Director of Federal Affairs, education, at the American Speech-Language-Hearing Association, shared "Our members, including audiologists, speech-language pathologists, audiology and speech-language pathologist assistants, and members of academia, found that by being able to provide services to students in the home environment, they could see some nuances about how the student learned." These encounters allowed specialists to observe students in real-world settings and helped caregivers feel more connected to their children's development These takeaways underscored a powerful truth: with the right support, virtual learning created new opportunities for families and school-based professionals to support student learning in new and helpful ways.

While educators worked heroically to adapt, many students with disabilities, particularly those from low-income, rural, or racially marginalized communities, faced some of the most profound disruptions to their learning (Crow, 2022; Dvorsky et al., 2023). Specialized services were harder to access, routines were overturned, and the loss of peer connection and in-person support took a deep toll. For many students, learning stalled. At home, caregivers stepped in to fill the gaps, often without the training, time, or tools they needed. The result was not just limited academic progress, but compounding stress for families already navigating significant challenges.

In the next section, we explore how K-12 and public health leaders can plan from the margins at the organizational level— that is, by examining how entire schools, districts, or systems identify gaps, allocate resources, and build partnerships to address inequities. Doing this work includes assessing which schools need the most support, understanding community-specific barriers to getting this support, and working across departments or agencies to deliver targeted, responsive solutions.

Planning from the Margins at the Organizational Level

While K-12 leaders plan from the margins at the individual level by considering the needs of students and families, planning at the organizational level means focusing on schools or organizations as a whole. Advancing equity requires knowing both the resources a school already has and the resources it needs. Similar to individual-level planning, understanding resource needs begins by asking the *right questions*—using tools like surveys, focus groups, interviews, listening sessions, or town halls. District leaders may be able to work with a university or community-based partners to document and analyze data to identify which schools are at the district's margins.

Leaders at Boston Public Schools (BPS), for instance, used multiple data sources to identify which schools and students were the most under-resourced. With about 45,000 students, BPS is home to 74% of Boston's school-age children. Nearly half of BPS students speak a language other than English at home, one in five has a disability, and half are economically disadvantaged (BPS, n.d.). Ensuring that every student has what they need to succeed—academically, physically, and emotionally— has long been a guiding commitment for the district. District leaders created BPS's opportunity index, for example, a mathematical formula that quantified access, to identify which schools and students are in most need of resources and then allocate resources. During the pandemic, BPS's commitment to equity and opportunity was tested. When concerns about ventilation and air quality emerged, the district combined data from multiple sources to guide an urgent and equitable response. To prioritize schools for indoor air quality improvements, BPS combined data collected from racial equity planning tools, the district's opportunity index, which identified underresourced schools and students, and data from new air quality monitors.

With these data in hand, Katherine Walsh, assistant director of planning, engineering, sustainability, and environment, and her team launched a district-wide air quality initiative. Instead of distributing resources evenly across schools, they prioritized buildings with the poorest air quality and the highest-need student populations. Walsh described it as a "thoughtful decision-making process to address air quality. We begin with why we are doing what we're doing, then consider how we will do it, who we will involve, and what are the potential equity impacts, both positive and negative."

Boston's data-driven equity-informed approach illustrates how school systems can use data to turn broad commitments into targeted action across entire systems. The Clark County School District (CCSD) in Nevada, the fifth-largest district in the United States, took a similar approach. Serving over 300,000 students across urban, suburban, and rural communities, CCSD used data to guide the delivery of health services in ways that reflected the geographic and economic diversity of the families it serves. For CCSD Chief Nurse Sheri McPartlin, ensuring that all families had access to the information and support they needed to stay healthy had been a top priority for almost 30 years. During the pandemic, McPartlin and her team translated that commitment into action by building systems that helped schools respond to students and families fairly and effectively. For example, McPartlin led the build-out of a centralized call center to manage illness reporting and track virus exposure for both students and staff. It was a major undertaking that responded to extraordinary demand—the center handled more than 15,000 calls each week at the height of the crisis.

In addition to the call center, CCSD's electronic medical record system enabled efficient case tracking and communication with families. CCSD's telehealth platform was also key to serving students' physical health needs and to controlling the spread of COVID-19. McPartlin stressed that strong partnerships made these initiatives possible, especially when it came to providing these resources to under-resourced schools. "Open communication with state and local public health agencies, along with collaboration with colleagues from other states through STAT calls," she explained, "helped shape our policies and gave us access to critical resources." STAT, introduced in Chapter 2, is a national action network that brings together state health departments to share resources and problem solve around pressing public health issues. The examples from Boston and Clark County show how equity-centered, data-driven and technology-based initiatives can protect entire school communities, attending to equity at the organizational level.

Another example of protecting students by working at the organizational level comes from Dr. Meagan Fitzpatrick, an infectious disease transmission modeler at the University of Maryland School of Medicine. She used advanced modeling to support equitable distribution of resources to schools during the pandemic. Modeling helps researchers forecast how a virus might spread by combining different data sources, ideally at the local level. Fitzpatrick and her team built simulations that mirrored the activity in real schools and household settings, then tested how different mitigation strategies, like masking, testing, and vaccination, might influence transmission of the virus. Fitzpatrick inputted local data into the models, such as absenteeism rates in high- and low-transmission areas, to predict how COVID-19 could spread under different conditions. These models helped identify which strategies were most effective at preventing school-based outbreaks. Reflecting on this work, Fitzpatrick explained:

> The main insight that our modeling work revealed is that schools can open safely if given the right tools and resources. We modeled in-school transmission, replicating the social structure inside school and at home. We found that schools are like mirrors: they do not generate high levels of infection when community incidence is low, but schools will amplify high transmission when it exists. If schools are given priority for rapid testing, vaccination, and improved ventilation, outbreak risk will decline. Unfortunately, during the COVID-19 pandemic, schools were not always prioritized for these resources.

Fitzpatrick's modeling made one thing clear: schools did not drive community transmission—they mirrored it. When local case rates surged, outbreaks in schools followed. However, as Fitzpatrick alluded to, testing sites opened first in corporate offices and commercial corridors, before they opened in schools. In addition to showing that schools reflected rather than drove transmission, her work underscored how schools were sidelined in some municipalities.

Planning from the Margins at the Community Level

At the community level, planning from the margins means identifying and addressing institutional, social, and political inequities that prevent people from achieving strong academic outcomes and attaining their highest level of health. The inequities that prevent strong health outcomes among students are referred to as social determinants of health. Social determinants of health are the conditions in which people are born, grow, go to school, work, and age. They are conditions over which individual people have limited control but conditions that significantly impact their health and quality of life. For example, forces like racism and intergenerational poverty can result in a parent with a lower-paying job with little to no time off. These jobs make it more logistically challenging, and often more costly, for parents to take their children to the doctor when needed, making it more difficult for them, than their affluent peers, to keep their child healthy and learning. Addressing social determinants means attending to the health disparities that accompany them. Health disparities are the preventable differences in disease, injury, violence, and access to opportunity that some populations experience more than others (CDC, 2024).

Reservations, border communities, and geographically isolated rural communities have fewer resources, less access to healthcare, and greater distances to travel for services and goods from grocery stores or medicines from pharmacies. For students of color, particularly Black, Indigenous, and Latinx students, the pandemic amplified long-standing disparities rooted in structural racism. These students were more likely to attend schools with fewer resources and more likely to be impacted by COVID-19–related illness and loss in their families and communities. Recognizing this broad spectrum of inequity is essential to understanding why planning from the margins is not just a strategy—it is a necessity.

Legacies of injustice do not exist in isolation. Instead, they are compounded by present-day economic and social conditions that continue to limit access to care. These layered inequities played out in real time in cities across the country, including New Orleans, Louisiana. In March 2020, just after Mardi Gras, New Orleans confirmed its first COVID-19 case. That spring, the city's death rate became the highest in the nation; 70% of those who died were Black residents, even though they made up only about one-third of the state's population (Zeller et al., 2021). New Orleans Public Schools sit within the city limits of New Orleans. The district serves approximately 43,000 students, over 75% of whom are Black and more than 85% of whom are economically disadvantaged. Many families in the district struggle to keep nutritious food at home and do not have reliable healthcare.

Dina Hasiotis McEvoy, the district's chief school support and improvement officer during the pandemic, led efforts to distribute technology, developed a roadmap to safely reopen schools citywide, and coordinated COVID-19 testing access for students and families. Hasiotis McEvoy recalls:

> We had to create as many partnerships as possible with our local health department and hospitals to bring testing into parts of the city that typically do not receive resources or support quickly. Eventually, we were able to offer testing, open to the community, at school sites, so that it was more widely accessible to all, which I think led to an increase in community trust and public safety.

Rather than waiting for help to arrive, the district brought services directly to the neighborhoods that needed them most—offering a model of community-based planning that put both urgency and access at the center. "Move fast and find your own solutions," Hasiotis McEvoy urged. "Don't wait for others to bring resources to you... and don't take no for an answer when you're fighting for those who are usually unheard." Socioeconomic inequities prevented families from accessing critical mitigation supports; understanding this at the community-level meant identifying and addressing these inequities instead of waiting for something to happen. Another powerful example of initiatives aimed at planning from the margins at the community level unfolded in Mississippi. Mississippi has 82 counties, the majority of which are designated as mental health professional shortage areas, meaning residents lack sufficient access to psychologists, psychiatrists, or licensed counselors. This issue became particularly urgent during the pandemic, when mental health challenges like isolation, anxiety, and depression surged.

In response, the Mississippi Department of Education partnered with the University of Mississippi Medical Center's (UMMC) Center for Telehealth to launch a statewide school-based mental health telehealth initiative in 2022. The program ensured that students in Mississippi's public schools had access to virtual medical services, dramatically shortening the time to access care. Where families once waited up to several months to see a medical professional, students could now speak with a counselor or nurse practitioner within a day or two of being referred. UMMC has become a national leader in telehealth, driven in part by the state's rural geography and need for virtual access. As Dr. Saurabh Chandra, chief telehealth officer at UMMC, explained,

> We have the responsibility not only for the patients within our facilities but for the health and well-being of the entire state. That mission, combined with our longstanding telehealth infrastructure, allowed us to quickly mobilize and meet the mental health and urgent care needs of schoolchildren across Mississippi.

As part of the initiative, schools were equipped with laptops and Bluetooth-enabled diagnostic tools—like digital stethoscopes and otoscopes—to support virtual urgent care visits with clinical providers. This initiative powerfully addressed geographic and socioeconomic inequities. Transportation challenges, time constraints, and limited financial resources became less predictive of students' access to care. This partnership between UMMC and the state department of education stands as a model for how states can innovate at the intersection of education, healthcare, and technology to reduce disparities at the community level.

Another example of addressing equity at the community level involves addressing state and federal regulations. During the pandemic, the STAT Network helped states rapidly expand school-based testing by sharing real-time innovations, like Texas's groundbreaking approach to CLIA waivers. CLIA waivers are federal certifications that allow non-laboratory settings, like schools, to perform simple diagnostic tests such as rapid antigen tests. Historically, CLIA waivers were granted on a site-by-site basis, a daunting challenge when there are hundreds or thousands of school buildings in a state. Texas, however, allowed K-12 schools to operate under an umbrella CLIA waiver, bypassing the need for each district to apply individually. After the director of Texas' K-12 school testing program shared this strategy on a STAT call, other states, including Massachusetts and Ohio, realized they could adopt the same statewide CLIA waiver method in their states. This collaborative knowledge-sharing was critical to scaling rapid testing in schools and keeping students safe in classrooms. These waivers allowed all schools in a given district to operate as testing sites, giving them the flexibility to identify cases quickly and keep students learning in person.

At the community level, delivering effective interventions requires more than good design. It requires understanding communities' capacity to implement the program well, with the necessary resources and personnel. When programs like school-based testing are rolled out without this awareness, they risk missing the very students and families who need support the most. During the pandemic, test-to-stay initiatives offered a clear example of how even thoughtfully designed strategies can fall short. Students who participated in a test-to-stay program were permitted to stay in school after exposure to COVID-19 if they agreed to regular testing. However, in districts without school-based testing, many students could not participate because testing sites were too far away or otherwise difficult to reach. For families without flexible jobs, reliable transportation, or paid leave, participating became nearly impossible. Instead of increasing access to in-person learning, the program left many students out. The lesson is clear: even well-intentioned programs to support schools during a public health crisis can deepen inequities if schools and districts lack the resources, infrastructure, or support needed to put them into practice.

▶ KEY APPROACHES TO PLAN FROM THE MARGINS

Creating the conditions for every student to learn, feel safe, and stay healthy is never simple—even under ideal circumstances. Two key approaches, however, can help K-12 and public health leaders do this work during crises: *prioritizing* the distribution of resources and *differentiating* supports. Prioritizing is about making decisions when supplies, funding, or staff are limited. Instead of allocating resources evenly, leaders look at where needs are greatest and direct support accordingly. Differentiating means customizing supports to meet the unique circumstances of each school or community, rather than assuming that one approach will work for everyone.

Both strategies start from the same place: acknowledging that public health crises affect communities differently. When leaders anticipate these differential impacts and plan with them in mind, they are better equipped to support those at the margins and keep all students safer, healthier, and more connected to learning.

Prioritizing Resources

During the pandemic, essential supplies—tests, masks, vaccines, even hand sanitizer—did not always meet demand. As shortages rippled through communities, the federal government, state agencies, and school districts had to make decisions

Prioritizing Resources	Differentiating Supports
• Use a recognized state formula • Use a recognized public health tool, such as the CDC's Social Vulnerability Index • Use locally collected data relevant to the issue, such as school-based vaccination rates	• Develop state policy that can be customized at the local level • Develop district policy that can be customized at the building level • Communicate in multiple ways to reach all stakeholder groups • Offer layered risk reduction approaches

Figure 3.2 Ways to Attend to Equity in Planning Interventions.

about where to send the limited resources available. Hannah Carter, project manager for school district environmental health at the Center for Green Schools, saw how thoughtful planning could shape those decisions. Working directly with K-12 leaders, she helped districts navigate indoor air quality improvements and prioritize investments when budgets were tight. "Aging infrastructure and limited funding meant that just dividing resources equally could leave the most vulnerable schools behind," Carter explained. "That doesn't happen when school districts leverage data on facility conditions, ventilation performance, and community vulnerability at the individual building-level to prioritize investments where there's the greatest risk."

Her insight on equity points to a key takeaway at the organizational level: when resources are scarce, data can guide tough decisions. By focusing on local conditions and acknowledging existing constraints, K-12 and public health leaders can target support where it is needed most. The following examples show how leaders in different states used data, from funding formulas to public health indices, to guide fair, timely, and effective resource distribution.

In the early months of launching a statewide school testing program, SHIELD Illinois faced a tough reality: there was not enough funding to include every K-12 district in the program. In the summer of 2020, a team of researchers from the University of Illinois Urbana-Champaign (UIUC), developed the covidSHIELD saliva test—participants would drool into a vial, and this PCR test could produce accurate results within 24 hours. Initially used within the university system, a number of partnerships across the state and an emergency authorization from the FDA meant that this simple, effective, highly sensitive, and specific test could be used in K-12 buildings. The SHIELD Illinois team worked with longstanding and trusted partners, including K-12 districts, the Governor's Office, the State Department of Health, the State Board of Education, and the Illinois Education Association to become one of the largest testing programs in the world. However, in the initial months, the team had to make difficult decisions about which districts to prioritize. Rather than build a new decision-making process from scratch, the team turned to a tool that school leaders across the state already knew well: Illinois's Evidence-Based Funding (EBF) formula.

In 2017, the EBF replaced Illinois's outdated "Foundation Formula," which had tied school funding to local property taxes. The older model left many property-poor districts chronically underfunded, while wealthier communities were able to contribute more dollars per student through their tax dollars. In contrast, the EBF required the state to fund districts based on a tiered system. Tiers are based on a formula that takes into account each local district's financial resources and the cost of educating all students, with additional funding granted based on the number of low-income students, English learners, and students with disabilities. Using the EBF tiers, the SHIELD team was able to quickly identify where operational and financial need was greatest and begin offering support to those districts. Their team helped with site setup, consent forms, staffing, training, and data reporting—tailoring each program to the district's needs. Because K-12 leaders were familiar with the tiers, districts could anticipate getting testing support (or not) before the initiative was funded state-wide.

While Illinois prioritized its testing rollout based on a school funding formula familiar to educators, Alabama's COVID-19 testing team took a different approach when faced with limited funds to launch its school-based testing incentive program. They turned to a trusted tool from the public health field, the Social Vulnerability Index (SVI), which ranks communities based on their capacity to prepare for and recover from public health threats. Developed by the CDC and the Agency for Toxic Substances and Disease Registry (ATSDR, 2024), the SVI uses U.S. Census data to rank communities based on 15 factors, including poverty rates, housing stability, transportation, and household composition. High SVI scores often reflect places where families face multiple, overlapping barriers: parents who cannot take time off work, limited access to health care, crowded housing, or unreliable transportation. By using the SVI, Alabama's team could identify which districts were most likely to struggle with the logistics of school-based testing and start there. Even though the tool was less familiar to education leaders than Illinois's school funding formula, it offered a practical, evidence-based way to guide early decisions.

While Alabama's team relied on a statewide index to guide resource distribution, districts like Jefferson County Public Schools (JCPS) in Louisville, Kentucky, used local data to prioritize where to allocate limited testing resources and nursing staff. In Louisville, local data offered a clear but concerning picture. The students least likely to be vaccinated were also missing the most school and falling behind academically. Many of these students attended the same handful of schools and lived in households with older or medically vulnerable family members—raising the stakes for any COVID-19 exposure. By following the school's internal health and academic data, JCPS prioritized schools with the most students at risk of experiencing serious consequences from COVID-19. Focused testing programs and school nurses assigned to these schools helped reduce spread, prevent disruption, and keep school a safer place to learn.

Across these examples, K-12 and public health leaders used data to prioritize where the risks were greatest and allocated resources to address those needs. Whether the resources were supplies, funding, or personnel, thoughtful planning helped leaders determine how to allocate what they had. In addition to directing resources first to under-resourced schools, leaders also had to ensure those resources were the right ones—matched to the specific needs of each community. Next, we explore how leaders put this principle into action—differentiating support so that every community received not just more resources, but the right ones.

Differentiating Resources

Differentiating supports means that states, school districts, and public health agencies can offer targeted and tiered supports based on specific school needs. Leaders in K-12 and public health know well: one-size-fits-all approaches do not work. This is where differentiation matters. Protecting school communities during a public health crisis requires tailoring strategies to fit local conditions. Each state, district, and community brings its own mix of cultural, economic, and logistical realities. What works in one may not succeed in another, even if each faces similar risks. To be effective, K-12 and public health leaders must deliver the *right* kind of support designed for each school and community's specific realities. This approach was adopted by practitioners across the country, including Dr. Christina Silcox, research director of digital health at the Duke-Margolis Center for Health Policy in Washington, DC, who developed national guidance on COVID-19 screening and diagnostics. While her work stressed the importance of clear and ongoing communication between public health officials, schools, students, and families, Silcox also recognized the importance of accounting for the specific characteristics of individual school settings and community values when selecting methods for mitigating risk in schools, rather than relying on the same solution for each building. This approach helped in "reducing spread and also building a community's trust that school was a safe place to be."

In Virginia Beach, Dr. Caitlin Pedati, public health district director, translated this concept—tailoring support to local needs – into action every day. Pedati described how effective pandemic responses required adapting what resources were distributed to which school buildings based on health data and the unique values and circumstances of each community. Whether driven by culture, infrastructure, or politics, every jurisdiction had its own rhythm and challenges. The work of adapting to that context, she noted, was best done locally— within the guardrails of the evidence-based guidance offered by federal and state partners. She shared, "communities and jurisdictions experienced COVID slightly differently, depending on the needs of that community or jurisdiction, depending on some of the mitigation measures that were used, depending on the interactions between public health and education." Her state, Virginia, is a commonwealth of geographic and cultural distinction: crabbers and watermen on the east, tobacco farmers in the south, the mountains of Appalachia to the west, and the political center of the country, the metro Washington, D.C. region, to the north. Virginia is also home to a large migrant community, with families following the crops and moving from district to district depending on the season. From the affluent capital suburbs to communities without running water or broadband internet, Virginians designate their state a commonwealth, highlighting the intention of its founders for power to reside in its localities.

To support effective outreach in this highly decentralized state, Joanna Pitts, School Health Nurse Consultant for the Virginia Department of Health, partnered with school nurses to design strategies tailored to each community's needs. When one school struggled to get more than 10% of families to consent to student vaccination, its school nurse stopped sending mass emails and instead started calling families directly. Those one-on-one conversations created opportunities for questions and conversation, building trust between families and the school. Consent rates climbed from 10% to 90%, a reminder that individual relationships still matter and that differentiating outreach to build on those individual relationships is essential.

IN BRIEF: STATE SCHOOL NURSE CONSULTANTS

A state school nurse consultant (SSNC) is a state-level role held by a registered nurse who supports K-12 districts on school health policies. They work with K-12 leaders around required vaccinations, related state and federal statutes, and specific individual health issues that a student has. They also answer questions from school nurses and K-12 administrators, and they serve as liaisons and advocates between school nurses and state policymakers.

Districts across the country tailored reopening strategies to meet the specific needs of their students and communities. For Chief Academic Officer Jeannine Medvedich at Chief Leschi Schools, this meant reopening in phases—starting with students receiving special education services during the winter of 2020–2021. By spring 2021, Medvedich reflected, "We couldn't push pause on kids' futures." To move forward safely, the district implemented a rotating hybrid schedule and adjusted supports based on what students needed most. They added plexiglass dividers for students who could not wear masks, set up outdoor classrooms to increase airflow, and used clear masks to ensure the youngest students, who were learning how to read, could see how their teachers' mouths moved during literacy instruction. Each of these decisions reflected a larger commitment to tailor supports to meet students' individual needs. Medvedich understood the urgency, exhorting, "Don't sit back and wait. Kids' lives are at stake. Education is the one thing that can't be taken away once you have it." She knew that they needed to find differentiated solutions so that students could be back in school safely.

Boston Public Schools (BPS) also differentiated as a way to address organizational-level inequities in indoor air quality. At the start of the pandemic, some buildings had central HVAC, some had steam heat plus limited mechanical ventilation, and some had steam heat with no mechanical ventilation. Buildings in the latter two categories, with steam heat, relied on working windows as their primary source of ventilation, and these buildings needed a different set of improvements than those with central HVAC. Drawing on technical guidance from the CDC, the Environmental Protection Agency (EPA), and the American Society of Heating, Refrigerating and Air-Conditioning Engineers (ASHRAE), the district implemented different strategies to improve air quality within each type of building. This approach ensured that buildings received the supports that worked with the type of ventilation in place. For example, some buildings received window air conditioning units. In buildings with HVAC systems, where allowable by the equipment, more than 4,300 filters were upgraded to MERV-13 filters. Across the district, 27,000 windows were inspected, and 12,000 were repaired.

However, providing different improvements to different school buildings meant difficult conversations explaining why those improvements did not look the same everywhere. When air filtration systems were installed in one building but not another, some families misinterpreted this as favoritism or neglect. It was not always clear to parents why certain buildings received upgrades before others, and it was hard not to wonder if their child's school had been overlooked. In reflecting back on these conversations, Walsh pointed out that transparency is not about saying what people want to hear. It is about being clear about the decision-making process and helping stakeholders understand the importance of differentiation, which is providing each building what it needs to be safe.

▶ RACIAL INEQUITY, LINGUISTIC DIVERSITY, AND COVID-19 HOSTILITY: THE CASE OF JEFFERSON COUNTY PUBLIC SCHOOLS, KENTUCKY

Race, class, and language are just a few of the social social determinants that shape students' lives both in and out of the classroom. These factors influence which school students attend, how their families engage with teachers, and the type of academic opportunities they can access. Beyond school walls, the same factors affect students' access to healthy food, medical and dental care, and the availability of safe spaces to play or spend time outdoors. In Jefferson County Public Schools (JCPS) in Louisville, KY, leaders were aware of disparities in testing and vaccination rates. These disparities did not begin with the pandemic, but the pandemic amplified them, confirming what JCPS leaders had long known about systemic inequities in their district.

This is a case about how a long-standing commitment to racial equity, shaped by local history and codified in district policy, helped guide JCPS's reopening during a time of crisis. This case offers a blueprint for how districts can act on that commitment in tangible ways—by prioritizing the distribution of resources to serve the areas of greatest need first, and by differentiating outreach and supports to respond to the different realities of each district community. JCPS's reopening story shows how equity-centered strategies can take shape at every level—from individual students, to entire schools, to the district and community as a whole.

Setting the Stage: A History Committed to Equity

JCPS is the largest school district in Kentucky and the 30th largest in the United States. Roughly 20% of families speak other languages in addition to English, and 63% of students are eligible for free or reduced-price lunch. In 1975, the Louisville school system—serving predominantly Black students in the city, and the Jefferson County school system, serving predominantly White students in the county—were court-ordered to merge following a landmark Supreme Court ruling on inter-district desegregation. Since that merger, JCPS's school board, along with district and school leaders, has worked to build a more inclusive and integrated public education system—one designed to serve students from a wide range of racial, cultural, and socio-economic backgrounds.

In the early 1980s, JCPS created its Diversity, Equity, and Poverty Division. This office helped formalize the district's commitment to addressing systemic inequities by providing targeted support for students from low-income households, advancing multicultural education, and developing tools to translate equity planning into meaningful action. In 2018, JCPS deepened that commitment by adopting its racial equity policy, with commitments to diversify the teaching staff and address achievement disparities, amongst other key goals (McLaren, 2018). This policy provided a framework for action, helping district leaders examine the potential impact of their decisions on historically underserved students and communities.

At the start of the pandemic, when schools closed and students shifted to virtual learning in JCPS, long-standing disparities, particularly around language, economic security, and digital connectivity, became more visible and more urgent. Linguistically diverse students, like their peers across the country, were more likely to live below the poverty line (Batalova & Fix, 2023; Charles et al., 2022), and less likely to have reliable internet, sufficient devices, or an adult available to support remote learning. Nearly half of the district's 96,000 students lacked consistent access to technology, leaving over 45,000 students disconnected from instruction and from opportunities to engage with peers and trusted adults. As COVID-19 magnified and accelerated existing inequities, district leaders began to develop reopening plans that centered equity by planning from the margins.

Navigating a Mitigation-Hostile Environment

During the pandemic, JCPS leaders made decisions in a politically charged, often contentious environment, where public health measures like masking, testing, and vaccines had become political flashpoints. By the fall of 2020, six months after the district closed its doors, JCPS was at the center of competing demands. The push to reopen came from all directions: families, business leaders, and political figures. While a vocal minority of parents called for a "return to normal," district leaders recognized that what had long been considered *normal* was shaped by deeply entrenched disparities.

Between 2020 and 2022, hostility toward public health safety measures gained traction. In 2021, Kentucky's legislature voted to strike down the statewide school mask mandate, overriding the governor's veto. Then in 2022, the state attorney general ruled that JCPS had violated state law by enforcing its own mask mandate during a school board meeting. Even though similar measures were in place in other districts across the state, the ruling only applied to JCPS; this raised questions about fairness and local authority. At the same time, the district faced two separate lawsuits challenging its masking and testing protocols. As JCPS developed its reopening plan, they did so within this politically charged environment. Despite intense political pressure, legal uncertainty, and parental divisions, district leaders kept student health and equitable access to learning at the center of their reopening plan.

Integrating Equity and Communicating with Families

With input from families, national experts, and organizations like the local chapter of the NAACP and the Louisville Urban League, JCPS examined how strategies such as school-based testing, masking, and physical distancing might affect different groups of students in different ways. Guided by their 2018 racial equity policy, district leaders used a standard set of guiding questions to shape decision-making including:

- *Which racial or ethnic groups might be disproportionately affected by this policy, and in what ways?*
- *What unintended consequences—racial or otherwise— could emerge?*

- *Have those most affected by the decision been meaningfully engaged in the discussion?*
- *What feedback did they share, and how was it incorporated?*

During these conversations, leaders heard from principals, educators, and staff that they needed support in helping students acculturate back to school, not just to classrooms, but to being in a social environment. Students were recovering from disconnection, grappling with food and housing insecurity, and, in some cases, experiencing and processing trauma. Recognizing the toll that isolation had taken on student's emotional development, JCPS temporarily paused suspensions for students in Pre-K through third grade, shifting the focus toward proactive, positive behavior strategies that prioritized growth over punishment. In addition, the district launched trauma-informed care training for educators and staff, and they hired and trained a full-time nurse for every school building.

These initiatives supported students when they were in school while families at home received regular updates about safety measures, school schedules, transportation, and other information that families needed to help keep their children safe and learning. The district mailed printed materials and emailed information to every household. However, many families preferred speaking over reading, and those without internet access could not always read emailed messages. Beyond this, reaching every family in a district where more than 150 languages were spoken required extra care and deliberate planning.

Because most nurses spoke only one or two languages, Dr. Eva Stone, JCPS's manager of district health, and her team relied on a telephone-based interpretation service to communicate with families, answering questions and addressing concerns about the district's soon-to-launch testing and vaccination programs. In addition, nurses and newly hired certified nurse assistants began meeting with families in person. They used each conversation as an opportunity to build trust and ensure families had the information they needed, in the language and format that worked best for them, to make informed health-related decisions.

Developing the Testing Program

A cornerstone of reopening was JCPS' school-based testing program—a program that was technically sound, manageable for school leaders, and accessible to families. Designing and delivering this program across the district's 155 school buildings required technical expertise, logistical coordination, and strong buy-in from district leaders, staff, and families. To develop its plan, JCPS leaders and their public health partners participated in the Cross-City Learning Group (CCLG, introduced in Chapter 1). They listened closely to what other districts were doing, such as how partners in New Orleans secured replacement test kits after a hurricane flooded their storage area, how partners from Tulsa vetted vendors for a data dashboard, and what it took for colleagues in D.C. to host their first drive-through testing event.

After every session, Stone began putting these strategies from colleagues across the country into practice. With support from the superintendent, Dr. Marty Pollio, and the school board, Stone and her colleagues launched a small-scale testing program for the district's in-person learning hubs, while schools across the district were still closed. These hubs provided in-person learning for students whose parents were essential workers and for students receiving special education services. District leaders visited the hubs and spoke directly with parents, students, and staff about rapid testing. They explained what testing entailed, how results would be handled, and why it mattered. Stone and her colleagues listened to concerns, fielded questions, asked the hub leaders and parents what would make testing work for them, and along the way, developed relationships with testing vendors, labs, and community-based organizations. As a result of these visits and the small-scale trials, and in conversation with families, staff, and nurses across the district, JCPS put their learning into practice at scale.

Faced with growing pressure and increasingly politicized debates over masking and testing, Stone and her colleagues kept their focus on what mattered most: building trust in the process and creating an effective and feasible testing program.

They concentrated on what they could control, such as increasing access to testing and communicating with clarity, consistency, and transparency. Early on, the district launched a public data dashboard that displayed up-to-date COVID-19 testing results across all schools. By making this data visible, JCPS sent a clear message: reopening decisions were being guided by data—and the health and safety of students and staff were the district's top priority.

The district also expanded testing access beyond school walls, establishing multiple drive-through sites to serve families and the broader community. When the Omicron variant swept through Louisville in late 2021, a program that had once collected just five samples per week rapidly scaled to collecting over 25,000. One partner described the shift as going from a "baby seal operation to a Navy SEAL operation." It was a striking transformation—and a testament to what deliberate planning, community trust, and cross-sector coordination could accomplish. JCPS's achievement evolved from a long-standing commitment to equity, listening to families and staff, a clear strategy for implementation, and strong partnerships, especially with the local health department, that were built over time.

Navigating Equity: Lessons from JCPS

For JCPS, the pursuit of equitable outcomes for all students was never an abstract principle—it was a lived commitment, grounded in the district's racial equity policy, supported by a legacy of community engagement and advocacy, and sustained through annual school-based equity planning. That policy set expectations for the district that supported equitable programs in classrooms, schools, and communities. During the pandemic, JCPS and its public health and community partners drew on this foundation to pursue health and academic equity in a time of crisis—they identified students at the margins, adapted supports to meet their needs, and stayed grounded in the day-to-day realities of school communities. The district's approach prioritized achieving equitable outcomes for all students at every level.

At the **individual level**, JCPS expanded virtual learning for medically vulnerable students, extended broadband access, and offered mental health services both online and in person. Leaders also communicated with families in accessible ways, in terms of language and format. At the same time, frontline staff, including bus drivers, custodians, nutrition workers, and substitute teachers, received long-overdue pay increases, in recognition of the essential roles they played in keeping schools safe and running.

At the **organizational level**, the district prioritized allocating investments that fostered safe and supportive learning environments to schools with the most vulnerable students first. They looked at data at the school-level to identify inequities and gaps and brought resources to schools with the greatest need. Throughout, communication was treated as essential infrastructure—not just a delivery mechanism, but a trust-building tool that aimed to meet families where they were.

At the **community level**, JCPS leaders used district-wide data to explore which social determinants of health, like poverty, were clustered in which schools.

JCPS leaders faced these inequities directly and took them into account as they planned. These efforts demonstrate how a long-standing, district-wide commitment to equity can translate into concrete actions that ensure that ensure all students have access to safe, in-person learning

In the next section, we offer a set of recommendations for leaders who want to *plan from the margins*—designing with, not just for, the students, families, and communities most often left out.

▶ CONSIDERATIONS FOR PLANNING FROM THE MARGINS

Throughout the pandemic, K-12 and public health leaders had to make fast, high-stakes decisions—often with limited resources and incomplete data. The most effective responses began with a commitment to supporting students and families who had long been overlooked and who and had less access to

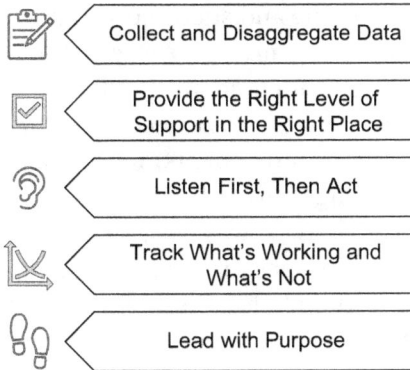

Figure 3.3 Considerations for Planning from the Margins.

essential health, education, and support services. The following actions can guide K-12 and public health leaders as they plan, implement, and assess school-based public health initiatives that center students and families at the margins.

Collect and Disaggregate Data

Aggregate data—data about sub-groups that are combined into one large group—can sometimes hide what is really going on. To understand who needs the most help, leaders need to break the data down, or disaggregate it—by income, language, neighborhood, attendance, vaccination rates, or other meaningful indicators. Several examples in this chapter show how state and local leaders used data to guide their decisions: SHIELD Illinois applied the state's evidence-based school funding formula; Alabama used the CDC's Social Vulnerability Index; JCPS tracked testing and vaccination rates by school. However, collecting and disaggregating data is not enough. What matters is what leaders do next.

Provide the Right Level of Support in the Right Place

Leaders can use disaggregated data as a guide to prioritize and differentiate resources and services so they are used as efficiently and as equitably as possible. A key principle to keep in mind is that equity does not mean equality. It means giving everyone what they need to be safe and successful. That looks different in every district—and sometimes in every school. Differentiating supports means that leaders identify different needs and then allocate resources to meet those needs. Giving every building the same air quality improvements, for example, is not useful when different buildings have different ventilation systems.

There is not one "correct" way to prioritize, but prioritization is most effective when decisions are driven by data and when leaders share the rationale for these decisions in a timely and transparent fashion.

Listen First, Then Act

K-12 and public health leaders need to ensure they share information with all families and community groups, while also listening to what these groups have to say. Effective communication is not just about broadcasting information—it is about listening, responding, and adapting. School nurses from Oregon to Kentucky to Florida did not simply hand out flyers or send out email blasts. They picked up the phone, asked questions, listened to concerns, and explained testing and vaccination options in ways that families felt were personal and respectful

How something is said—and who says it— especially in multilingual and multicultural communities, can matter as much as the message itself. K-12 and public health leaders attended to the language and communication preferences of communities, and they listened to what stakeholders had to say. When leaders see that certain stakeholder groups are not engaging in safety measures, taking the time to figure out how to initiate and maintain communication is key.

Track What's Working and What's Not

Good intentions do not guarantee good results. Leaders need to know whether their strategies are working—where, and for whom. That means planning for evaluation from the start of a new program or initiative. This might mean starting with a small pilot, like JCPS's initial testing program, that allows leaders to spot gaps early and make changes before scaling up. It also might involve leaders on the ground where initiatives are happening, talking with impacted stakeholder groups to understand their experiences.

Planning with evaluation in mind ensures that leaders, funders, and the school community know the extent to which an intervention achieves outcomes of interest. Evaluation findings can help decision-makers know if they are using limited time and resources judiciously. Importantly, monitoring and evaluating programs can help ensure that new disparities have not been created or that existing disparities have not gotten worse. It is also critical that program planners, implementers, evaluators, and participants have dedicated time to reflect on learnings throughout program delivery, so they can understand what to keep doing, what to stop doing, and what to change.

Lead with Purpose

Advancing equity is not easy. Planning from the margins often involves prioritizing resources, changing routines, or challenging how things have been done. Not everyone will cheer for those changes, and some may try to undermine them. Stakeholders who had been doing well under prior initiatives might push back against new plans that upset the status quo; they might also push back against plans that give the appearance of negatively impacting them or their children, even if it is in appearance only.

In the face of pushback, K-12 and public health leaders need to stay focused on their goals and develop strategies to communicate about their strategy. In many parts of the United States, for a variety of reasons, it is not easy to pursue initiatives aimed at increasing equity, in education or public health. Having a clear focus and internal and external supports to stay committed are requirements for ensuring greater equity for students on the margins.

▶ PUTTING EQUITY AT THE CENTER: COMMUNICATING DIFFICULT MESSAGES

To build trust and take action to advance equity, leaders also need to communicate clearly, consistently, and strategically.

REFLECTIONS FROM THE FIELD: PRESERVING DIGNITY, SAFETY, AND HOPE

Aníbal Soler, Jr. served as superintendent of Schenectady City Schools in Albany, NY during the pandemic. As superintendent, she worked to ensure that all students in this racially diverse district continue to learn and thrive, acknowledging that the role of the district during the crisis extended beyond academics.

During the COVID-19 pandemic, leading a school district in New York meant prioritizing equity and trust in every decision. We prioritized transparent communication and community partnerships to ensure our most vulnerable students had access to learning, meals, and mental health supports. What was hardest—and most important—was recognizing that our response wasn't just about academics; it was about preserving dignity, safety, and hope for every child and family during difficult and unpredictable times.

From equity, we turn next to communication. During a public health crisis, effective communication allows partners to share information with students, staff, families and the broader community so everyone has a shared understanding of risks, how to protect themselves and each other, and what to expect next.

References

Agency for Toxic Substances and Disease Registry. (2024). Social vulnerability index. Retrieved from https://www.atsdr.cdc.gov/place-health/php/svi/index.html

Batalova, J., & Fix, M. (2023). *Understanding poverty declines among immigrants*. Migration Policy Institute. Retrieved from https://www.migrationpolicy.org/sites/default/files/publications/mpi-poverty-declines-immigrants-2023_final.pdf

Boston Public Schools (BPS). (n.d.). Data and reports. Retrieved from https://www.bostonpublicschools.org/about-bps/data-and-reports?utm

Bronfenbrenner, U. (1977). Toward an experimental ecology of human development. *American Psychologist, 32*(7), 513.

Centers for Disease Control and Prevention. (2024). What is health equity? Retrieved from https://www.cdc.gov/health-disparities-hiv-std-tb-hepatitis/about/index.html

Charles, R., Collyer, S., & Wimer, C. (2022). The role of government transfers in the Black-White child poverty gap. *Poverty and Social Policy Brief, 6*(3). New York: Center on Poverty and Social Policy, Columbia University.

Crow, O. (2022). Education inequality during COVID-19: How remote learning is widening the achievement gap and spurring the need for judicial intevention. *BCL Review, 63*, 713.

Dvorsky, M. R., Shroff, D., Bonds, W. B. L., Steinberg, A., Breaux, R., & Becker, S. P. (2023). Impacts of COVID-19 on the school experience of children and adolescents with special educational needs and disabilities. *Current Opinion in Psychology, 52*, 101635. doi: 10.1016/j.copsyc.2023.101635

McLaren, M. (2018). JCPS approves 'historic' policy to tackle racial inequity. *Courier Journal.* https://www.courier-journal.com/story/news/education/2018/05/09/jcps-racial-equity-policy-achievement-gap/593270002/

Rose, D. H., & Meyer, A., with colleagues at CAST. (2002). *Teaching every student in the digital age: Universal design for learning.* Alexandria, VA: Association for Supervision and Curriculum Development (ASCD).

Turk, M. A., Landes, S. D., Formica, M. K., & Goss, K. D. (2020). Intellectual and developmental disability and COVID-19 case-fatality trends: TriNetX analysis. *Disability and Health Journal, 13*(3), 100942.

Zeller, M., Gangavarapu, K., Anderson, C., Smither, A. R., Vanchiere, J. A., Rose, R.,... & Andersen, K. G. (2021). Emergence of an early SARS-CoV-2 epidemic in the United States. *Cell, 184*(19), 4939–4952.

Chapter 4

Communicating Clearly in Chaotic Times

> We know that teachers trust principals, and families trust teachers. We needed to craft the messages we were going to send to ensure that administrators understand and can train up teachers, so that teachers can share up-to-date info when they're in the grocery store, when they chat with their neighbors. If public health can get us the correct information, we can help with that cadence and clarity of communication.
>
> Tracy Jentz, (former) Communications and Community Engagement Coordinator, Grand Forks Public Schools, North Dakota Vice President, National School Public Relations Association

Schools closed for summer break in 2020, leaving educators, students, and families with one urgent, unanswered question: *Will they open in the fall?* Without clear or immediate answers from official sources, many turned to social media, television, and word of mouth. The media, both traditional and social, quickly became an unofficial mediator, shaping public understanding of what was happening, why, and what to do next (Anderson, 2007). However, these platforms also became vectors for confusion and harm. Misleading health information minimized the severity of the virus, cast doubt on public health guidance, and contributed to mistrust and division, costing countless lives in the process.

DOI: 10.4324/9781003608844-4

As inaccurate health information ran rampant, K-12 and public health leaders worked in partnership to develop communication plans to counter these messages. As Jentz's reflection makes clear, district leaders in Grand Forks, North Dakota, recognized the role of trust in communication and the power of trusted messengers early on. In her district, Jentz ensured that teachers had access to clear, accurate information that they could pass along to students in classrooms and to families in grocery store aisles and during neighborhood conversations.

For teachers to be trusted public health messengers, school systems need to work *with* public health, not simply to receive information, but to translate it, coordinate it, and deliver it in ways that resonate with the communities they serve.

In this chapter, we turn to the third principle of our framework: communication. By situating communication within trust and equity, we show how it can become more than just messaging—it can be a strategy for increasing safety, connection, and public confidence. We begin by describing key features of effective communication that K-12 and public health leaders can use to communicate with each other and with their stakeholders. This approach to communication is multidirectional, coordinated, transparent, and evidence-based. Through real-world examples, we explore how these features have been put into action and examine some of the common challenges leaders have faced. We then turn to Aurora Public Schools in Colorado, a district where students and families speak more than 160 languages and where public opinion was deeply divided over mitigation efforts. In closing, we offer a set of recommendations for how K-12 and public health leaders can establish a shared approach to communication, both in advance of and during a public health crisis.

IN BRIEF: MISINFORMATION AND DISINFORMATION

In the context of a public health crisis, *misinformation* refers to inaccurate health information that is spread during the emergency. This information is not backed by scientific evidence. *Disinformation* goes a step further: it is intentionally false or misleading content spread to manipulate, deceive, or influence people's beliefs or actions (Nagar et al., 2024). Both misinformation and disinformation can erode public trust by minimizing the severity of a virus and casting doubt on public health guidance. When this happens, evidence-based responses can be undermined, and mistrust can spread.

When K-12 and public health leaders share evidence-based information through trusted messengers and networks, they support families in making informed health decisions. Joanna Pitts, the school nurse consultant in Virginia, emphasized the importance of respect and trust in school communication. "Validate what families' concerns are," she said, "and be able to respond with an evidence base coming from a trusted partner." Evidence-based information refers to facts or guidance that are backed by high-quality research, data, or expert consensus rather than personal opinion or speculation. When a school nurse is seen as a credible messenger and is equipped with reliable information, families are more open to listening and engaging in conversation. When this happens, school–family communication becomes more effective and meaningful. The same principle applies to communication between K-12 and public health partners. When relationships are built on trust, and everyone has an equitable opportunity to engage in conversation, partners have confidence that the information and knowledge they share with each other is valid and reliable.

▶ WHAT MAKES COMMUNICATION EFFECTIVE

Communication is not just about sharing facts. It is a way to build stronger, more trusting relationships between schools, public health partners, and the communities they serve. As effective leaders develop formal communication plans or informally communicate with stakeholders, they strive to make sure that all stakeholders have access to communication streams, both to receive accurate information and to share their questions, concerns, or experiences. The following features reflect what leaders on the ground shared in reflecting on their communication practices.

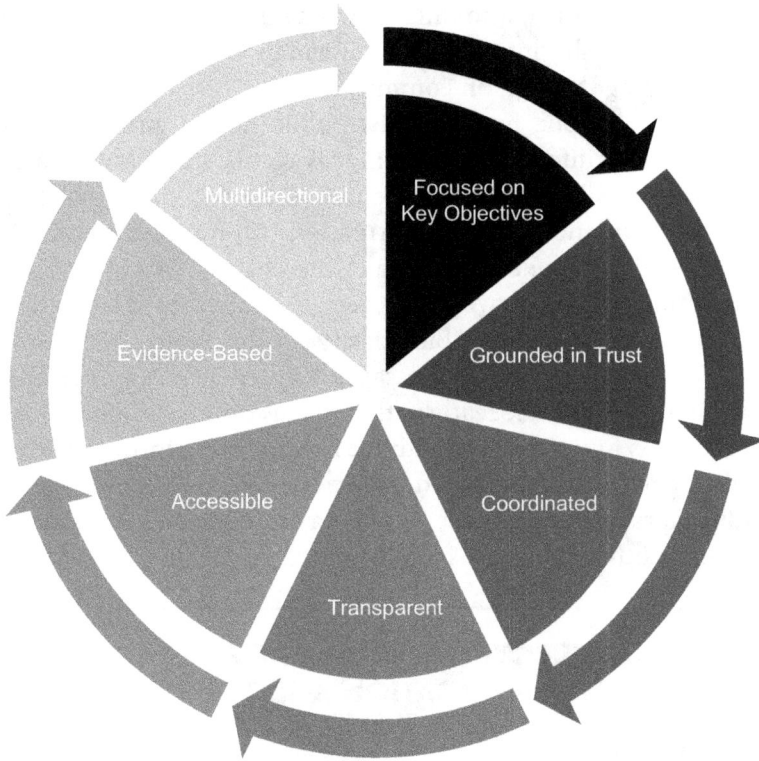

Figure 4.1 Features of Communication.

▶ COMMUNICATION IS GROUNDED IN TRUSTING RELATIONSHIPS

In K-12 and public health partnerships, trust makes effective communication possible. When trust is present between individuals and institutions, communication becomes a connection. Marlee (Kingsley) Carlos, founder and CEO of a leadership consulting firm, underscored this point, reflecting that

The steps taken today to build trust and understanding increase the speed and efficacy of decision-making when crises occur. The ability to coordinate communication effectively during any crisis is strongly influenced by the interactions that take place well before anyone knows a crisis will occur.

In practice, trust in communication means that partners believe each other is sharing accurate information, listening openly, and following through on commitments.

During a public health crisis, public health guidance will change as new information becomes available. Inaccurate health information will circulate as the public tries to make sense of changing guidance, and disinformation will be spread by individuals trying to take advantage of the chaos. When there is a foundation of trust between partners, they are able to freely discuss concerns, raise questions, clarify confusion, and collaboratively develop coordinated messages that reflect accurate health information. Of all the features that make communication effective, trust is foundational. Without it, accurate information can be disregarded, questions and honest conversations never occur, and leaders lose the chance to build a strategic plan that leverages each other's strengths and resources.

REFLECTIONS FROM THE FIELD: COMMUNICATION AND TRUST

Elizabeth Coke, acting deputy of the Emergency Preparedness and Response Branch of the Centers for Disease Control and Prevention, found communication to be essential to her partnership work as it led to increased trust and effective program implementation.

> Coordinated communication and trust are essential components of collaboration between public health and K-12 schools. During the COVID-19 response, our team worked diligently to share accurate and transparent information, fostering trust among administrators, educators, parents, and students. By collaborating across various educational settings, we ensured that all students and families received the necessary resources and support to make informed decisions. Working side by side with education and public health partners enabled us to effectively implement public health initiatives, enhancing our preparedness efforts.

Trusted Messengers Help Reach Diverse Stakeholders

Trusted messengers play a crucial role when it comes to community trust in public health guidance. Trusted messengers are individuals who already have the confidence of a particular group, who work with districts or public health organizations to deliver health-related information. The concept is not new. In the 1990s, public health campaigns trained respected community figures to model and promote healthy behaviors within their social networks (Kelly, 2004). During the pandemic, trusted messengers included pediatricians, faith leaders, celebrities, teachers, school nurses, and even students. They worked alongside K-12 leaders and local health departments to share timely information about vaccines, testing, masking, and more. Importantly, the role of trusted messenger is context- and message-dependent. Who is trusted in one community may not be seen as a trusted messenger in other communities, and individuals trusted to share certain messages may not be as trusted with other types of messages.

Trusted messengers showed up in unexpected and meaningful ways across the country. In California's San Gabriel Unified School District, lead district nurse Kathy León partnered with Dr. Daniel Soto, assistant professor at the University of Southern California's Keck School of Medicine. Soto recruited over 20 graduate students to support K-12 student connection and implementation of COVID-19 mitigation strategies in Los Angeles County districts, including in San Gabriel Unified School District, which serves approximately 4,600 students. The graduate students, many just a few years older than the high schoolers, quickly became relatable role models. They provided hands-on support to students during a critical time, and they also provided a glimpse of what students might aspire to in their own educational journeys.

The graduate students also listened. At a time when students were navigating not just the uncertainty of COVID-19, but a host of personal and social challenges, having someone who would simply listen mattered. The graduate students became trusted adults, close enough in age to feel relatable, but steady and knowledgeable enough to offer support. These relationships helped students feel seen and supported. "These relationships weren't built by talking about COVID-19," León explained. "They were built by learning about each other—supporting each other. That kind of connection created the trust we needed to talk about testing and vaccination when the time came."

Still, when graduate students suggested ways to strengthen school-based mitigation efforts in the districts, conversations with K-12 leaders occasionally faltered. As Soto reflected, "Many public health practitioners don't 'speak school,' and many K-12 leaders don't 'speak public health.'" This language gap often slowed down communication at precisely the moments when efficiency was critical. To keep initiatives on track, Soto and León learned to center their communication around terms like "access" and "all students"—language that emphasized shared priorities and helped sidestep political tension. In many settings, those terms moved conversations forward more effectively than words like "equity," enabling partners to stay focused on their goals.

In addition to graduate students, León looked to teachers as trusted messengers in the work she did with vaccination clinics. She brought in teachers—not to give vaccines, but to sit with children throughout the process. León felt that

> this is someone that the child knows and feels comfortable with. When you're doing something that is not comfortable, like getting a shot, they have some familiarity and someone to trust. At the same time, teachers are someone that students and families will talk with, they will ask questions.

Identifying messengers who are trusted often means taking into consideration who the messenger is and how they are connected to the intended stakeholder group. For León, the professional role of teacher was one that connected to students, while for Soto, the professional role and language of academia initially disconnected him from schools, while the youth of graduate students helped them to connect with high school students. It is useful for leaders to consider how a messenger's professional identity, such as job or formal role, as well as their personal identity, such as their age, race, or gender, might inform how they communicate with others. This does not mean that leaders or messengers' identities must "match" those of stakeholder groups, but that these identities can inform how messages are heard. Being aware of one's own identity helps leaders approach others with respect and empathy. When leaders reflect on how they are being received by a stakeholder and when they ask stakeholders what they can do differently, they are able to communicate more effectively.

REFLECTIONS FROM THE FIELD: MAKING GUIDANCE ACCESSIBLE AND FAMILIAR

Morgan Ripski, consultant and testing coordinator with New Orleans Public Schools in Louisiana, involved medical advisors in her regular meetings with district personnel in order to increase access to and understanding of changing guidance.

> As COVID testing coordinator for NOLA Public Schools, I led a city-wide effort to provide free weekly testing for every public school student. We built trust through consistent communication—biweekly calls with school nurses and operations leads, and immediate updates when protocols changed. We included medical advisors on every call, making expert guidance accessible and familiar. Every frontline staffer had my direct number and used it. Building a tight, responsive team—and showing up consistently—proved to be the single most important factor in earning the trust of those doing the hardest work on the ground.

Communication Travels Strategically in All Directions

Multidirectional communication between partners flows in all directions. It moves horizontally across institutions at the same level—between schools in a district or among local public agencies—and vertically, as information, concerns, and decisions move between school sites and district offices, and between local districts and state agencies. K-12 and public health partners share information, raise questions, and learn from one another. Emily Frank, associate professor with the University of California, San Francisco, highlights this point, reflecting that "The COVID pandemic revealed our natural tendency to exist within silos. It quickly became clear that there was an immense need for cross-sector listening and understanding before truly effective planning could take place and protocols could be successfully implemented."

Two-way communication between K-12 leaders and families is especially important during a crisis. When K-12 leaders communicate *with* families—instead of *at* them—decisions about next steps are more likely to reflect families' realities, priorities, and concerns. Those whose voices had been on the margins are moved into the conversation. When families can see how their perspectives have shaped decisions, they are more likely to trust the effort and continue to engage in conversations with the district. Because of this, communication is participatory and inclusive. It requires that K-12 administrators, public health leaders, and families actively exchange ideas, offer feedback, and create a culture where open dialogue is encouraged. This kind of communication values listening as much as speaking and creates space for everyone to share experiences, raise concerns, and shape decisions—regardless of their position or title.

One state health department in the southwest embraced a multidirectional approach as it worked to support local health departments and K-12 districts during a time of intense pressure and resistance to safety measures. The state health department hired a former physical education teacher, someone who understood schools from the inside, to deliver public health guidance to educators, school boards, and superintendents across the state. As this former teacher traveled the state, he did more than share information—he listened. He asked school leaders and community members what was feasible, what was working, and where guidance was falling short. He also facilitated weekly conversations with local health departments. Then he brought all of that feedback back to the state health department. In doing so, he helped both public health and education leaders "hear each other's language."

This did not guarantee that everyone agreed or that behaviors changed overnight. But his approach set a new tone. It modeled curiosity, respect, and humility. Over time, it reshaped how K-12 leaders viewed their relationship with the state health department. By prioritizing listening, he helped set a norm for how trust could grow between systems. As he put it: "People understand and know when their voice is being valued and listened to." When that happens, communication helps to forge a relationship, one that increases the likelihood that, in the next crisis, public health messages will be heard, considered, and acted on.

Equally important is making sure that messages not only travel strategically in all directions but also resonate with the people they are intended for, ensuring equity in communication. That is where thoughtful delivery becomes critical. Brandi O'Brien, manager of programs and development with Utah Physicians for a Healthy Environment, saw this firsthand while helping distribute HEPA air purifiers to schools across Utah. She shared that

> messaging had to be carefully curated for each audience, and finding the right people to talk to within school systems and public health departments was often a challenge. It was a reminder that trust, especially in public health, takes time and intention to build.

Her experience underscored how even well-intended messages can miss the mark if they are not tailored to the audience, context, and channels that communities already know and trust. What seems like the clearest, most unified message to an organization can fall flat if it is shared in a format families cannot access, in a language they do not read, or through channels they do not trust.

Leaders in Grand Forks Public Schools in North Dakota learned this as well. Jentz and her team realized that families were not responding to voicemails, emails, or phone calls and therefore not getting critical updates about mitigation strategies and school reopening plans. Rather than continuing with more of the same, they pivoted. "We found that text messages were being read within five minutes over 95% of the time," Jentz explained. Her team adopted special software to translate and send text messages into multiple languages and embedded links to the district's newsletter in every text message. "We found that was a really effective way to get information out to our families. The text messages became a lifeline for us when some of those other communication platforms were not working." Jentz's experience highlights that a communication strategy requires intentional decisions about accessibility, delivery, and form. The form of communication—whether a text message, flyer, press conference, or social media post—can vary depending on the audience and the platforms they trust and use.

Partners Benefit from Coordinating Their Messages

While the form or language can vary, the function and content of the message remains the same: to equip families with clear, consistent information they can understand and use. When school districts, public health departments, and other partners share different messages or emphasize different priorities, it creates confusion and erodes trust. Especially when public health guidance evolves, coordination ensures that messages reinforce each other, helping families make informed decisions with confidence.

When K-12 leaders and public health partners plan a communication strategy together, deciding what to say, how to say it, who should deliver it, and how, their messages are more likely to stick. That means people are more likely to remember those messages—and use them to make decisions that protect themselves and their families. This is especially true when public health guidance is translated into plain language, shared in accessible formats, and delivered by people and through platforms families already know and trust.

REFLECTIONS FROM THE FIELD: THE POWER OF COMMUNICATION

Ann Covey, education associate with School Health Services and state school nurse consultant at the Delaware Department of Education, emphasized the value of communication and collaboration.

Delaware's Community of Practice was vital in ensuring coordinated, equitable public health support across schools. By fostering real-time collaboration between the Department of Education and Department of Public Health, this initiative enabled timely updates on CDC guidance and mitigation strategies. A key lesson learned was the power of consistent, open communication—through virtual office hours for school nurses and a CDC Foundation–funded liaison team—building trust and streamlining care coordination. This ongoing collaboration has strengthened public and school health infrastructure, ensuring resources, guidance, and standards of practice reflect school community needs and promote health equity.

Coordinated messaging across institutions strengthens the message. In Illinois, Dr. Brian Wegley, superintendent of the Glenview Northbrook District 30 during the pandemic and now retired, knew how important it was to reach all stakeholders through channels that they trusted. This was thanks, in part, to partnering with Cathy Kedjidjian, the executive director of communications and strategic planning in a neighboring district, and also the president of the National School Public Relations Association (NSPRA) at the time.

The suburban district has a student enrollment of about 1,250 and serves families who speak more than 60 languages at home; a quarter of students come from low-income households. Just before the pandemic hit, the district had been preparing for a referendum (a local vote about increasing taxes to support schools) and had already invested in broad outreach. Wegley shared, "We had set up a great deal of community engagement to make sure that we were reaching people" and continued:

> But we had to double down on that. Our translators and interpreters—we really had to rely on them, even more heavily than we already had. We had to ensure that our website, which is ADA compliant, has translation tools and other accessibility tools. We had to make sure that we were utilizing our website as a tool, as a hub. Before the pandemic no one ever said, 'I cannot wait to go home and look at the school website,' but during the pandemic, that really was the hub.

In addition, with support from their local government, both Wegley and Kedjidjian served on a local Coronavirus Response Task Force, which allowed them to "stay in step" on messaging. They created communications together, translated messages, and disseminated them at the same time through all district and governmental communication channels. Wegley reflected that "the decisions of the schools impacted our park districts and libraries and vice versa. Consistent responses across all of our agencies were essential."

IN BRIEF: MAKING COMMUNICATION ACCESSIBLE

The federal Americans with Disabilities Act (ADA) requires that public schools, and all Title II entities, communicate messages in ways that are accessible to individuals with communication disabilities, such as those related to vision, hearing, or speech. According to the ADA, "The goal is to ensure that communication with people with these disabilities is equally effective as communication with people without disabilities." Importantly, the ADA (2020) notes that this communication must be multidirectional, and communicators must attend to how individuals both receive and convey information. K-12 and public health communication meets this requirement when leaders think about different aspects of how messages are sent, including the complexity of the message, the larger context of the communication, and the individual's preferred format for communicating.

The National Center on Health, Physical Activity and Disability (n.d.) offers specific strategies for communication, such as providing alternative text (alt text) descriptions of images, paying attention to color contrast in image design, and including captions and transcripts with videos. The Center also includes tips for creating presentations and a checklist that can be used to assess accessibility.

Dr. Heidi Schumacher, who led the pandemic response for District of Columbia Public Schools (DCPS), also identified the importance of coordinating messages. She shared that "our strength as policymakers, community leaders, and front-line practitioners lies within our ability to leverage our relationships, to be clear and consistent in our communication, and to meet communities where they are." Whether through interpreters, translated websites, or multilingual texts, K-12 and public health leaders in these districts had a shared goal to ensure that a single message was accessible to and resonated with many constituents. That kind of coordination made it more likely that families would stay informed, connected, and protected.

Developing a Shared Message Through Coordination

In cross-sector collaboration and during times of political division, identifying a specific goal can help partners develop a shared message. In the fall of 2020, as the FDA prepared to authorize COVID-19 vaccines for youth ages 16 and older, Christie Scott was already thinking ahead. As acting director of community relations for Fairfax County Public Schools, a suburban district just outside Washington, D.C., with more than 180,000 students and over 12,000 staff, she knew the district would need a focused communication strategy to support vaccination. Scott and her team wanted to keep the message simple, direct, and centered on what families cared most about. "We basically looked at the landscape in our community," Scott explained.

> We wanted to find a mutual point we could agree on regarding the issue of vaccination. From the school system, from parents, families, teachers, and other staff—the one thing everyone could agree on is that we want kids safely learning in classrooms. So, we kept our vaccination messaging narrowed in on that. The whole time. We didn't get into any of the other stuff that was not our conversation to have. We simply talked about vaccination as a tool to keep your children safe and learning in person, which is what we all want. That helped us avoid having to get into [other] conversations. We were not engaging in a debate.

Scott's approach illustrates the value of narrowing in on a single, shared objective. When partners begin with agreement on the *why*, they are better positioned to communicate the *what*— even when the broader landscape is noisy or contentious. Finding that shared objective can take time and conversation. As one public health modeler shared, agreeing on shared goals is often the hardest part, but a critical starting point. "It's important to ask what do we ultimately want to accomplish and for whom and by when? What are our objectives around attendance policies, objectives around protecting vulnerable families… what are our community objectives?"

When partners take the time to name and agree to objectives, they reduce confusion and hone their communication. Irma Snopek, Policy and Communications Director with the Illinois State Board of Education, put it simply: "All of those challenging decisions were made easier because we had a North Star to follow." A clear objective—a North Star—helps teams draw boundaries around the conversation. People may still hold a range of views, but they can work together toward the clear objective that they identified together. SHIELD Illinois, introduced in Chapter 3, brought together local and state government leaders, educators, public health experts, and unions. Audrey Soglin, former executive director of the Illinois Education Association, recalled how complex the work of message alignment was:

> We put out joint statements as a team. We did not always agree at the outset; we ironed it out as a team, not in front of the public. We had to be very careful about what we shared with stakeholders. We didn't want to throw anyone under the bus. There were tense moments as we developed unified messages, with six organizations, six communications directors, and six general counsels. It wasn't easy—it took a lot of perseverance and collaboration. But if you're committed to getting it done, it will get done.

The consistency of SHIELD's messaging was the result of ongoing meetings into the late hours of the night and early hours of the morning between multiple organizations, including labor and government. Snopek reported that "once we agreed that the goal was to reduce transmission while continuing to provide an environment where students could learn, the conversations focused on what prevention strategies were appropriate to achieve that goal."

Sometimes, the opportunity for coordination arrives unexpectedly. In March 2020, as the COVID-19 crisis was just beginning in the United States, members of the National School Public Relations Association (NSPRA) were gathered for their regional meeting. During the conference, Michigan Governor Gretchen Whitmer announced that all public schools in the state would close. The timing was abrupt—but the gathering offered a rare chance to act quickly and together. Karen Heath, director of communications for the Berrien Regional Education Service Agency in Michigan, and meeting coordinator, worked with her colleagues and immediately shifted gears. Jentz, who led communications and community engagement for her district in North Dakota, attended the meeting and recalled what happened next:

> We stopped the conference and had a statewide writing session. We had the best brains in the room, and we felt that if we had one letter for all districts—if we all brought back to each of our districts one message, and we shared it at the same time and on the same day—if families all got one message, this would help families understand.

Instead of returning to their districts with different messaging, communications leaders returned to their districts with one unified message, helping school communities navigate an uncertain moment with a little more clarity and a lot more coordination. Dr. Greg Holzman, former state medical officer with the Montana Department of Public Health and Human Services, highlights the importance of commitment to a shared goal when schools, communities, and public health work together.

> Schools are among the most potent and vital partners in building safe and healthy communities. The best public health plans will not succeed—public health cannot happen—by one person or even one organization but must be with the commitment and work of the entire community.

Effective Communicators Share What They Know—Even When They Don't Know Everything

Effective communication is transparent. This means leaders are clear about how decisions are made, even during a fast-moving public health crisis filled with uncertainty. Throughout the pandemic, K-12 leaders showed transparency and built trust by developing and sharing public health guidance from local, state, and federal agencies, and by grounding their decisions in available data. Heather Drummond, who served as the testing branch manager for the COVID-19 Response at the Washington State Department of Health, explained how this approach shaped her team's efforts to scale school-based testing across the state:

> Supporting school testing during the pandemic response demonstrated how important transparency and communication are to foster trust quickly and prompt collaborative decision-making. We were able to build strong connections that we wouldn't have otherwise thought about if we were coming up with solutions on our own.

Transparency does not require having all the answers—but it does require being open about what is known, what is not known, and how decisions are made. During the pandemic, K-12 and public health partners who communicated early and often about available data, like community transmission rates, school-based case counts, and vaccine eligibility, helped build trust. Even when data were incomplete or rapidly changing—for example, as scientists worked to understand new variants or assess how well different mitigation strategies were working—leaders who shared what they knew, and what they were still learning, signaled honesty and accountability.

By being upfront that guidance might evolve as new evidence came in, leaders created space for action, built relationships, and kept the public informed. Mary C. Wall, former chief of staff of the White House COVID-19 Response Team, emphasized the importance of walking people through that process:

> We were all subject to an evolving virus and continued to be subject to this evolving force that kept throwing different challenges to us. It was very important to be upfront and show our work, showing how we got to the point of making a decision, and being really clear about what parameters we were balancing as part of the decision-making process.

Sharing the "why" behind decisions—especially when guidance changed—helped K-12 and public health leaders communicate more effectively, even while acknowledging uncertainty.

Acknowledging what is *not yet known* is also a vital part of transparency. Many leaders earned trust by being honest with each other about what they did and did not know. Dr. Jennifer Lepard, chief of Health, Wellness and Community Partnerships at the Oklahoma State Department of Education during the pandemic, described how conversations with her state-level peers looked in practice:

> These were very private conversations, very frank. It was a lot of us talking about what we were worried about, what we were scared about, what we each knew, and what we did not know. These conversations formed a bond between us, a professional friendship, built on this foundation of trust and vulnerability.

K-12 leaders can extend that same transparency to families. Letting families know that answers are still emerging, promising to follow up when information changes, and noting that information *will* likely change, can foster reassurance and respect. In Grand Forks Public Schools, Jentz and her team made this a cornerstone of their work: "We don't know yet, but we'll get back to you when we do," was, in her words, "the fuel to be successful in the face of another day of uncertainty." This kind of open, ongoing communication helps people manage uncertainty. "Uncertainty is not the best place to be," explained Dr. Julia Fraustino, associate professor of strategic communication and director of the Public Interest Communication Research Laboratory at West Virginia University in Morgantown. She continued,

> We either want to take some kind of action to alleviate that uncertainty, or we want to run away and hide to avoid it. So, in uncertain times, one way to provide reassurance, even if you don't have all the information, is to offer clear, consistent, and actionable communication.

While transparency builds trust, it also builds momentum. When K-12 and public health leaders are honest about what they know, what is uncertain, and what people can do next, they move from just informing the public to equipping them. One of the most powerful tools for doing that is data—not just shared, but translated, contextualized, and made meaningful.

Using Data for Decisions Grounds Communication

Thoughtful data sharing is central to transparency as a key feature of communication. This often involves publicly accessible data dashboards with current data. However, during the pandemic, not every district had a strong data infrastructure. Without clear, accessible tools, families were left guessing about risk—and leaders struggled to make timely decisions. "Our goal was to get Tulsa, Oklahoma students back to school and their parents back to work," said Jenna Grant, then resource development manager for the Tulsa Health Department and its nonprofit branch, Pathways to Health. With resources from the local health department, Jennifer Harper, a public health consultant, worked with Tulsa Public Schools to develop and launch a COVID-19 dashboard to help families and staff track local trends and make informed choices about masking, testing, and school operations. The dashboard was simple but effective. It was updated regularly and designed for use on mobile phones. (See Appendix F for tips on building a data dashboard.) Grant credited her community of practice, the Cross-City Learning Group (CCLG), with helping Tulsa access expertise and tools beyond its local reach. "In a small city in Oklahoma," she explained, "you don't always get expert resources." The CCLG connected the team to national peers, technical assistance, and proven strategies for developing and hosting a data dashboard, making it possible to translate data into action at the local level and help get students back to school.

Virginia's approach to data transparency during the pandemic was not just a best practice—it was state law. In January 2022, legislation was passed requiring all healthcare providers who administer vaccines to participate in the Virginia Immunization Information System (VIIS), a statewide vaccine registry. Around the same time, the state also required the Virginia Department of Health (VDH) to create a public-facing dashboard to track COVID-19 outbreaks. Like many public health surveillance tools, the dashboard relied on regular data submissions from local health departments, schools, and medical providers. Joanna Pitts, school health nurse consultant with the VDH, played a central role in making public health data accessible during the pandemic, and designed dashboards with families, school nurses, and district administrators in mind. "We wanted everyone to be able to follow our vaccination progress," Pitts explained. "Creating something accessible and giving folks information in real time was part of our mission to promote the COVID vaccine." These dashboards presented key information in a simple, visual format that could be easily understood and used. With just a few clicks, users could see how vaccination efforts were going in their school, helping families decide what steps to take to protect their children—and giving school leaders concrete data to guide their outreach.

What made data-sharing especially effective was how VDH partnered with the Virginia Department of Education (VDOE) to ensure that data were usable, timely, and accessible to all stakeholders. Each week, VDH and VDOE co-hosted virtual meetings with school nurses and nurse coordinators across the state. They shared the latest guidance on vaccine safety and eligibility, reviewed the newest dashboard data, and helped school health staff craft clear messages for their communities. These regular check-ins gave school nurses the tools—and confidence—to talk about vaccination in ways that felt relevant to the students, families, and educators they served.

The easy to use and up-to-date dashboard gave families the information they needed to make their own decisions, and increased their trust in, and reliance on state agency resources. It also strengthened trust between local districts and state agencies by providing a shared resource to guide reopening, vaccination strategies, and family communication.

Project: ACE-IT (Assuring COVID Education through Intensive Testing) is another example of how a team used data visualizations and clear, accessible language to support district leaders when they made decisions about reopening and safety protocols. The project was a groundbreaking and far-reaching collaboration across five counties in Southeastern Pennsylvania initiated in the fall of 2020 with the PolicyLab at Children's Hospital of Philadelphia (CHOP). The project was the nation's first large-scale school-based testing program using newly developed rapid antigen tests. At the heart of the project was a simple goal: keep schools open by decreasing transmission of the virus from person to person. To achieve this goal, the team took a two-pronged approach: first, they tested asymptomatic individuals to catch individuals who were unknowingly spreading the virus. Then, they used modeling to predict what could happen if key behaviors and every-day practices changed, like the percentage of students who masked, the number of feet that desks were spaced apart, and whether people at restaurants ate indoors or outdoors.

The project team worked hand in hand with local public health agencies, intermediate units, and school districts to get testing off the ground, prioritize the most vulnerable students and staff, and ensure individual districts and schools retained autonomy by overseeing their own implementation of the school-based testing program.

From the outset, the project team built a communication strategy based on trust and transparency, ensuring that families and school leaders could see the data itself, the models that projected different outcomes, and the assumptions that shaped those models. Project Leaders chose to share everything, and they translated that complex information into public-facing dashboards, maps, and blog posts that made the science understandable and actionable. One team member reflected,

> Number A versus Number B is less important than the messages we are communicating to people about what different models mean. We invested a lot in our communication strategy because we needed to provide output that was interpretable to parents, schools, and policymakers. It wasn't going to be enough just to do those scientific models.

The team worked to make the science visible and meaningful to parents and educators, illustrating how interventions like masking and limiting indoor dining could slow transmission. As a result of this highly collaborative, cross-sector work, schools had data-based alternatives to full lockdowns. Those with strong prevention strategies, including asymptomatic testing, masking and distancing became "islands of safety in a sea of transmission", as one team member put it. ACE-IT's modeling work helped shape national policy. The team demonstrated how interventions could slow transmission. It also demonstrated how quickly trust and infrastructure could be built when partners align around a shared goal, use timely data to guide decisions, and communicate clearly across systems and with the public. The project highlighted the power of distributed leadership and school-level flexibility, showing what it takes to move from science to real-world implementation.

Using Evidence-Based Health Information to Counter Falsehoods

In a crisis, people want quick answers to urgent questions. However, during the pandemic, scientific understanding about the virus was still evolving. As researchers learned more about transmission, infection risks, and prevention strategies, the public health guidance that communities received also evolved. If leaders wait for "perfect" data, inaccurate health information can take hold. K-12 and public health leaders learned this the hard way when they faced an overwhelming flood of both accurate and false information from digital and physical sources. Recognizing how a swell of contradictory information could create confusion the World Health Organization labeled this phenomenon an "infodemic" (WHO, 2021). As Nagar et al. (2024) note, one of the best ways to stop inaccurate health information from taking hold is to preempt it by sharing evidence-based messages.

K-12 leaders can work with their public health partners to set up systems to identify inaccurate health information, and then they need to decide how, and if, they respond. Social listening is one approach that leaders can use to identify inaccurate information that is spreading within a community (Stewart & Arnold, 2018). This approach involves paying attention to conversations and questions across stakeholder groups, by following conversations in comment sections of an online newspaper or noting the questions asked during town halls or through call centers. In Oregon, Wisconsin, social listening did not just happen online— it happened through conversations. Superintendent Bergstrom, introduced in Chapter 2, recalled how, during the height of the pandemic, parents regularly reached out with questions about things they had seen or read. "Parents would send me medical articles," she said, "and ask me, 'What do you think about that?'" Some suspected the information was not accurate and were looking for confirmation from someone they trusted. Others simply wanted to understand how their schools were responding. Instead of dismissing these concerns or answering them herself, Bergstrom drew on her strong relationships with local public health partners and medical experts from the University of Wisconsin. Together, they made sure that families received factual information, grounded in the latest guidance. In that moment, social listening helped school leaders understand family concerns early, respond with care, and reinforce community trust. Because the district, university, and health department were aligned, families heard one message—from multiple credible sources—and could make informed decisions with confidence.

Still, not every rumor needs a response. At times, it may be easy to spot "trolls"—someone who is posting messages on social media platforms for the goal of being offensive or provocative; at other times, however, inaccurate health information may be packaged in such a way that it looks realistic, drawing on images or charts and appealing to people's emotions. Partners can look to their shared objective and messages to determine if they should respond or not, rather than using limited time and resources to address every rumor. At Chief Leschi Schools, the Tribal Council and district leadership stayed focused on a shared message that COVID-19 is a medical emergency. "We didn't allow the tail to wag the dog," said Chief Academic Officer Medvedich. Her team chose to not respond to every conspiracy theory, social media rumor, or angry phone call. Instead, with the support of their Tribal Council, they stayed grounded in science and recommendations from the state's public health guidance. They focused on protecting their students and staff through consistent, fact-based messaging.

K-12 and public health leaders face difficult choices about how to respond to inaccurate health information. Researchers from John Hopkins University (Nagar et al., 2024) developed a useful guide to help organizations decide if they should respond. The first factor to consider is the seriousness of a rumor and the likelihood that community members, or specific groups, might believe it. For example, families that already used Hydroxychloroquine for its intended use, to treat rheumatoid arthritis, might be more likely to believe that this drug could treat or prevent COVID-19, which is inaccurate. Another factor to consider is an organization's capacity to respond. To assess K-12 and public health partners' capacity to address inaccurate health information, they need to assess their own resources, including people with subject matter expertise and trusted relationships with communities, as well as the financial and material resources to develop and disseminate an effective response. A third factor to consider is the potential unintended consequences of responding. Depending on the specific rumor, responding might create mistrust between leaders and communities.

In a high-stakes crisis, choosing not to respond is a choice. This is not to argue that leaders should never respond to rumors, but in situations where inaccurate health information abounds, leaders need to respond with intentionality. When K-12 and public health leaders respond with intention, grounded in shared goals, trusted relationships, and clear communication, they are more likely to be heard, believed, and trusted.

▶ NAVIGATING COMMUNICATION AND TRUST ACROSS LANGUAGES: THE CASE OF AURORA PUBLIC SCHOOLS, COLORADO

Aurora Public Schools (APS), also known as the Adams-Arapahoe School District 28J, is one of the most culturally and linguistically diverse districts in the western United States. Located just outside Denver, APS serves 40,000 students, 75% of whom qualify for free or reduced-price lunch. District families speak more than 160 languages, and communities in the western part of the district tend to have lower incomes and less access to essentials like transportation, medical care, healthy food, and clothing than their more affluent peers in the southeastern region.

As the pandemic entered its second year in the winter of 2021, public health clinics and private medical facilities across the country were at or near capacity and lacked the human resources to support vaccine administration, creating the need for schools to get involved (National Association of County and

City Health Officials, 2023). At this time, families in the district had mixed feelings about mitigation measures but shared a common goal: they wanted students back in classrooms. Dr. Marnie McKercher, APS's school health administrator, focused her messaging on that shared goal. Like her nurse leader colleagues around the United States, she promoted vaccination as the fastest and safest path to a return to in-person learning.

Because so many families spoke languages other than English, the district had to find ways to communicate clearly, consistently, and inclusively. McKercher needed to understand what families needed and also needed to find a way to do this with limited staff. Despite being the fifth-largest district in the state and located in a healthcare-rich area, APS had only a small team of school nurses and was regularly overwhelmed by demand for health-related services even before the pandemic. McKercher and her team gathered feedback through in-person parent presentations and discussions at both the school and district levels, and by using online surveys. "Parents shared what they needed to know, what questions they had about COVID in general," she explained, "including what the district was doing to keep students healthy and reduce risk of illness."

To communicate across language, McKercher's team started by translating key information about COVID-19 and school-located vaccination events into the ten most frequently spoken languages in the district. "Once we found our rhythm with the top ten languages," McKercher noted, "the translation team identified they could scale up to 25 languages. It took us about four months to scale up—a monster job for the translation team because we were constantly updating the health guidance in these documents." The district also created prerecorded voice messages in 25 languages, with details about vaccination events and updates on changing mitigation policies. "School nurses and family liaisons notified us if there was a request for a specific language, and we would submit it to translation services," said McKercher. McKercher reflected, "I wish we would have had capacity to do more", underscoring both the demand for multilingual communication and the district's commitment to meeting families where they were.

Creating Space for Two-Way Communication

In-person town halls with live interpretation gave families an opportunity to ask questions and gave the district an opportunity to listen. APS paid for interpreters to translate in real-time, and families used headsets connected to microphones. "APS has a parent advocacy group with multiple cultures and languages represented," McKercher explained. "They requested live Q&A sessions with live translation." She also met with religious leaders and regularly collaborated with the APS Newcomer Team, which worked closely with families that were new to the United States.

As the community slowly began to trust the messages that were shared by the district, McKercher was invited to speak at local meetings. These events, she said, became "invaluable to understanding what families needed, and to feel confident that we were sending messages out and providing resources that were responsive to those needs." Some families emerged as trusted messengers themselves, especially immigrant families from war-affected regions or refugee camps who were already familiar with the dangers of infectious disease. These families helped spread fact-based information about vaccines and played a critical role in boosting confidence. "At first it was a trickle," McKercher said, "but once we got some buy-in in the community—it really took fire."

Addressing Concerns with Hosting Vaccination Events

Even with growing support, launching vaccination events at APS schools was not easy. Leaders were wary of political backlash, especially amid national and local tensions around vaccines and masking. To ease internal concerns, McKercher began referring to vaccination events as "school-located" rather than "school-hosted" vaccinations, a subtle shift that signaled principals did not need to "own" the event; they only needed to provide the space. Early events went smoothly, and hesitation among school leaders began to subside. School nurses became frontline champions for these efforts. They helped coordinate logistics and hosted weekly learning sessions to stay coordinated on the messages they shared with families and the various supports, like home visits, they were providing

Still, tensions persisted. At one of the first vaccination event, an anonymous caller threatened violence, accusing the district of "killing children." When police were called in, their presence raised additional fears among undocumented families, many of whom worried they would be asked to show identification. In response, APS reassured families that no documentation would be required, and vaccine providers were instructed not to ask for any. To reinforce the protocol, APS began to include a clear disclaimer on every event listing, stating that no identification or documentation would be required. "We posted this information at the top of our webpage," McKercher explained, "and required all providers to include the same message on their event registration pages. No vaccination event was promoted without making that absolutely clear."

Despite these hurdles, the events were packed. At one early site, people were so eager to get vaccinated that they nearly drove over barricades to get in. "Apologizing for the long wait times turned out to be a bigger concern than the threatening phone calls," McKercher recalled. "It was essential that the event take place when and where it was advertised." This type of consistency and reliability built trust, and trust was key to getting people through the door.

Developing New Partnerships

Throughout the district's response, McKercher focused on listening. She made a habit of asking colleagues across departments, "What do you know?"—a question that led to new partnerships and brought fresh insight into different stakeholders' experiences. One such partnership formed with the Family Engagement Department. Through school-based family liaisons, staff who had long-standing relationships with families, the district was able to gather information about concerns, rumors, and community needs. Working together, the health services and family engagement teams co-authored messages that were clear, accessible, and grounded in both science and community priorities. "We kept our information at an accessible reading level," McKercher said. "We had a clear message that vaccinating will get students back into schools." By combining their knowledge and deep community relationships, these teams helped translate public health guidance into messages families could trust and act on.

▶ COMMUNICATING WITH PURPOSE THROUGH PARTNERSHIP: LESSONS FROM AURORA

In Aurora Public Schools, communication was not always perfect, but it was consistent, thoughtful, and rooted in partnership. McKercher and her team sent out frequent messages, often repeating key information, but few families felt overwhelmed. In fact, most welcomed the steady updates. Families wanted to know what was happening, and they trusted the district more when communication was consistent and accessible.

Importantly, communication did not just flow one way. APS leaders created space for families to ask questions, raise concerns, and offer input. That multidirectional approach helped the district focus on what mattered most to families: keeping kids safe and learning in person. Instead of getting pulled into political debates, APS stuck to a clear, shared message—delivered in multiple languages, and through multiple formats, so every family had access to the same critical information.

McKercher's leadership was central, but she did not work alone. Strong relationships across departments and with local public health agencies turned a challenging task into a shared mission. Together, they built a coordinated approach that reflected a deep understanding of family needs and helped unify the community around the common goal to increase vaccination and keep schools open.

▶ CONSIDERATIONS FOR ESTABLISHING EFFECTIVE COMMUNICATION

Effective communication across institutions and stakeholder groups takes work, but it is a critical part of building strong partnerships. Next, we outline practical strategies that K-12 and public health leaders can use to communicate more effectively during a crisis and beyond.

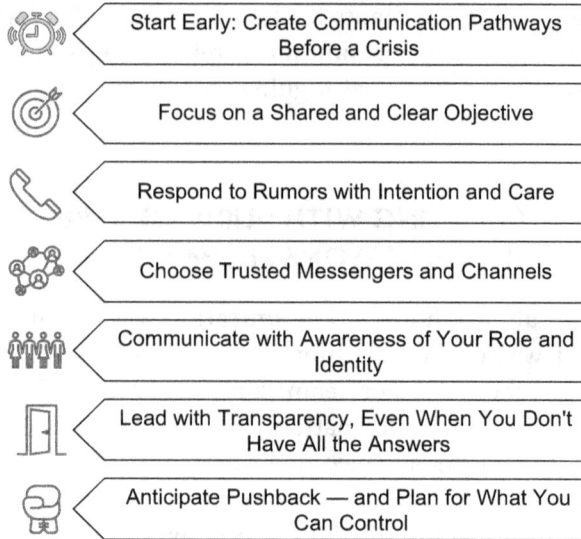

Figure 4.2 Considerations for Effective Communication.

Start Early: Create Communication Pathways Before a Crisis

When families see public health as a partner, an ally in keeping their children safe and healthy, they are more likely to listen during a crisis. By connecting early and often, schools and public health partners can build relationships that matter long before the next emergency arrives.

Part of this involves making public health visible. K-12 leaders can support this by spotlighting their partnerships with public health during "ordinary" times. Joint initiatives around youth violence prevention, mental health, or routine vaccinations can be powerful starting points. Clear, consistent communication about how the work helps students lays the groundwork for trust in public health partners that can hold steady when facing a public health crisis.

Focus on a Shared and Clear Objective

It is easier to align a message when everyone shares a similar view of the problem, but that is not always realistic. K-12 and public health partnerships often bring together people with different experiences, priorities, and beliefs. Instead of striving to agree on everything, strong partnerships focus on finding common ground—a clear, targeted objective that everyone can rally around.

For example, if the shared goal is reducing COVID-19 transmission, partners can concentrate on what levels of transmission are acceptable for their schools and community. That conversation may still be difficult, but it narrows the scope, keeps attention on what matters most, and avoids getting sidetracked by unrelated issues. Once partners identify a shared objective, they can reinforce it through clear communication, repeating key messages, and connecting each decision back to the central goal.

Respond to Inaccurate Health Information with Intention and Care

In a crisis, one thing is predictable: rumors spread fast. Without clear, timely guidance from trusted sources, people often latch onto whatever information is most available, even if it is wrong. We saw this repeatedly during the pandemic. That's why we encourage K-12 and public health partners to communicate clearly and early, even when answers are still unfolding. Sharing reliable information as soon as it is available, acknowledging that the situation is still evolving, and assuring families that accurate guidance is on the way can stop inaccurate health information from gaining traction. When community members have been swept up in false narratives, leaders benefit when addressing stakeholder concerns and offering accurate information from trusted sources. When leaders communicate with empathy and clarity, they create space for people to pause, reflect, and reconnect with the facts. And the more clarity leaders provide, the less room there is for confusion to grow.

When rumors do surface, it is important to remember that not all of them require a response. Addressing every piece of inaccurate health information and responding to social media trolls distract from organizations' core priorities. Instead, leaders should focus on delivering consistent messages tied to their stated goals. That focus helps communities stay centered on what matters most. To avoid reacting impulsively to every rumor, leaders can establish clear criteria for when and how to respond (e.g. Nagar et al., 2024).

Choose Trusted Messengers and Channels

Who delivers a message matters. Trust looks different in different communities, and K-12 and public health leaders need to think carefully about who families are most likely to listen to and what platforms they are most likely to use. Public health messages often ask people to do something new, like get vaccinated or wear a mask. This type of guidance is more likely to be effective when it comes from someone who shares the community's values and speaks their language—literally, culturally, and metaphorically. Leaders can strengthen their messaging by involving families and community stakeholders in the design, translation, and delivery of communication.

Once a message is out, it is important to assess how people are responding to it. Leaders can track reach and engagement using social media analytics, by following local discussion boards, or by simply asking community members what they are hearing. Feedback loops help fine-tune communication and build trust over time.

Communicate with Awareness of Your Role and Identity

Understanding where you come from—your job title or role, your experiences, your cultural identity—is essential when building trust, especially in times of crisis. Every individual brings a unique perspective shaped by their lived experiences, a concept referred to as positionality. Positionality influences how we understand others and how they understand us.

Leaders who are aware of their positionality are better equipped to earn trust, such as those who recognize they represent historically privileged institutions. They acknowledge the harm institutions like theirs have caused, such as the U.S. Public Health Service's Tuskegee Syphilis Study. This awareness shapes how they approach partnerships, with humility and a willingness to listen first.

Lead with Transparency, Even When You Don't Have All the Answers

In times of crisis, people naturally look to leaders for answers. But no one has all the answers—especially in a fast-moving public health emergency. Rather than pretend otherwise, strong leaders name what they know, what they do not know, and what they are still learning. This kind of transparency builds credibility, which builds trust. K-12 leaders are not public health experts, and they acknowledge this by inviting public health partners into the conversation. Asking questions, sharing concerns, and developing guidance with medical professionals is a sign of strength and leadership. In any public health crisis, scientific understanding will evolve. New evidence may lead to new recommendations, and abrupt changes can feel unsettling. Being transparent about that process can help families anticipate shifts without losing confidence in the system.

Transparency also means sharing the data behind decisions. Dashboards are one way to do this—especially when they are built with the public in mind. In places where public health mandates were limited or absent, timely, localized data helped individuals make informed decisions. Clear, accessible data do not just answer questions; they show that schools and public health agencies are committed to openness, partnership, and public safety.

Anticipate Pushback—and Plan for What You Can Control

One of the most important ways K-12 and public health leaders can strengthen their communication strategy is by preparing for disagreement before it arises. Leaders should expect—and plan for—the fact that some guidance will be questioned or rejected, especially when fueled by inaccurate health information. At times during a crisis, K-12 and public health leaders will receive intense negative press and threats. They may attend local school board and health board meetings with angry stakeholders arguing for or against different proposals. Focusing on their sphere of influence—rather than getting stuck in frustration over what they cannot control—is known in clinical psychology as *radical acceptance* (Linehan, 1993). Practicing this means acknowledging reality as it is—that guidance will change and families will be frustrated. This kind of acceptance does not mean leaders agree with what is happening, or that they stop trying to improve things. It means they do not fight what they cannot control and instead focus their energy into responding—clearly, constructively, and in partnership with others.

Putting It All Together: Trust, Equity, and Communication

Effective communication is about listening as much as speaking, making sure information is accurate and timely, and ensuring that all stakeholders are part of the process. This kind of communication only works when trust and equity are present, as trust, equity, and communication are deeply intertwined. Communication rooted in trust is more likely to be heard, and communication grounded in equity ensures that information is linguistically accessible and culturally relevant. Communication designed in partnership can move communities from confusion to clarity, from fear to action.

Throughout the pandemic, we saw how communication could become a bridge or a barrier. When communication flowed with intention and clarity, it brought people together. When it faltered, inaccurate health information and fear rushed in to fill the silence. When K-12 and public health leaders communicated with humility, respect, and purpose, they built stronger partnerships and stronger communities.

As K-12 and public health leaders continue their work together, through this pandemic and beyond, these lessons remain essential. When they communicate clearly, act collaboratively, and center the needs of the most vulnerable, they do not just keep schools safe. They help create communities where every student and family is informed, supported, and included.

References

Americans with Disabilities Act. (2020). ADA Requirements: Effective Communication. Retrieved from https://www.ada.gov/resources/effective-communication/

Anderson, G. L. (2007). Media's impact on educational policies and practices: Political spectacle and social control. *Peabody Journal of Education, 82*(1), 103–120.

Kelly, J. A. (2004). Popular opinion leaders and HIV prevention peer education: Resolving discrepant findings, and implications for the development of effective community programmes. *AIDS Care, 16*(2), 139–150.

Linehan, M. M. (1993). *Cognitive-behavioral treatment of borderline personality disorder.* New York, NY: The Guilford Press.

Nagar, A., Grégoire, V., Sundelson, A., O'Donnell-Pazderka, E., Jamison, A. M., & Sell, T. K. (2024). *Practical playbook for addressing health misinformation.* Baltimore: Johns Hopkins Center for Health Security.

National Association of County and City Health Officials. (2023). NACCHO's School-located vaccination clinic toolkit. Retrieved from https://www.naccho.org/programs/community-health/infectious-disease/immunization/tool-school-located-vaccination-immunization

National Center on Health, Physical Activity and Disability. (n.d.). Best Practices for Accessible Communications. Retrieved from https://www.nchpad.org/resources/best-practices-for-accessible-and-inclusive-communications/

Stewart, M. C., & Arnold, C. L. (2018). Defining social listening: Recognizing an emerging dimension of listening. *International Journal of Listening, 32*(2), 85–100.

World Health Organization. Infodemic. 2021. Available from: https://www.who.int/health-topics/infodemic#tab=tab_1

Conclusion

Preparing Leaders for What the Future Brings

Over the previous chapters, we have shared stories of how different districts partnered with local and state public health departments, connected with peer networks, the private sector, and university researchers for support and brainstorming, and worked to build or repair trust with a range of stakeholder groups. As the country worked to bring students back to buildings, as schools became testing and vaccination sites, and as new and changing data continued to surface and guidance evolved, leaders emerged, ready to navigate the educational and health challenges brought by the COVID-19 pandemic.

This book has argued that three commitments—trust, equity, and communication—formed the foundation of effective school–public health partnerships during the pandemic. We developed this framework by listening to the voices of K-12 and public health leaders as they reflected on their work to reopen schools during a global health pandemic. This framework highlights the critical role of **trust** between partners at the individual and institutional level, a shared commitment to advancing **equity** demonstrated by deploying strategies to increase positive academic and health outcomes for all students, and multidirectional, transparent, and accessible **communication** to enable both trusting relationships and actions that center the needs of those on the margins. These principles are interdependent and synergistic. When they are leveraged, they can create

DOI: 10.4324/9781003608844-5

conditions that support academic achievement and the health and well-being of students and staff. When leaders engage in these practices and hone these skills *before* a crisis occurs, their leadership skills *in the face of* crisis are practiced and routine.

▶ LOOKING BACK TO GO AHEAD

In the previous three chapters, we illustrated how leaders put the principles of this framework into practice. We reflected on the critical role of relational and institutional trust—between K-12 leaders and public health partners, and between both groups and the communities they serve. We emphasized the value of initiatives that meet communities where they are, and how "listening before leading" helped rebuild trust where mistrust had taken root, even during times of fear and confusion. We examined how shared understandings of equity anchored and focused response strategies, and we explored how sharing fact-based communication, to convey rather than to convince informed families and demonstrated respect for their ability to make decisions independently. This approach to building and leveraging partnerships —grounded in trust, equity, and communication— likely saved countless lives during COVID-19, and made meaningful differences in the experiences of students, staff, families, and communities.

In this chapter, as we look to the future, we begin by recapping key insights from leaders who put the principles of the partnership framework—trust, equity, and communication— into action. We then consider how K–12 leaders can adopt a public health mindset that recognizes their role as leaders in keeping students safe with cross-sector partners. We conclude with guidance on how partnerships can be built before a crisis so that leaders are better prepared for what comes next.

▶ KEY INSIGHTS

A commitment to *trust* is more critical than ever. Rebuilding trust is one of the most urgent challenges facing schools and public health today. Confidence in public institutions— including schools and public health agencies—has been in decline for decades, with sharper drops since the pandemic began (Leslie, 2023; Merod, 2022). In 1974, 54% of respondents to NORC's General Social Survey reported "a great deal of confidence" in those running public health institutions. By 2021, that number had dropped to just 38%. The implications are real: during a public health crisis, reduced trust means fewer people are willing to follow guidance from local or national health authorities and fewer lawmakers support that guidance through policies, mandates, and funding.

Trust in K-12 leadership means that parents and community members will reach out to schools during a crisis, sparking cooperation and constructive discussion. While trust in a school might begin with respect and regard for a teacher or principal, it can expand to trust in the organization's collective actions. K-12 leaders' trust in public health institutions at the local and state level means that they are better positioned to work together to achieve meaningful, measurable, and sustainable changes in students' health and wellness. These positive outcomes in turn, can build trust in public health recommendations during a crisis among school community members.

A shared commitment to *equity* will help partners develop a clear vision of what equitable health and academic outcomes look like—and how to get there. Those strategies are most effective when they are informed by all stakeholders and bounded by shared values like fairness, kindness, and empathy. To develop or refine a strategy, shape evaluation efforts, and ensure initiatives do not exacerbate pre-existing inequities, leaders can reflect on the following questions:

- What groups will be the most affected?
- What barriers need to be addressed?
- What assumptions are we making?
- Whose voices are not at the table?
- How will we know that what we're doing is working?

Partners in trusted relationships can ask each other difficult questions about access and equity with the goal of helping the partnership achieve its objectives. Issues of access, race, and social class, in particular, can be difficult topics to discuss in constructive ways, and trust lays a foundation for conversation.

Without trust, people may be wary of asking questions that might be interpreted as blame, and important questions are then never discussed or addressed. Finally, a commitment to *communication* that is multidirectional and transparent helps partnerships thrive. Effective communication is not just about sending messages—it is about making sure they are heard and trusted by all stakeholders. That means paying attention to language, literacy, and culture. It also means taking the time to understand the communication norms and values of different groups, identifying trusted media channels and messengers, and assessing whether or not messages are resonating. K-12 and public health leaders can rely on trained professionals and community-based experts who translate complex public health information into plain language that families can understand.

Strong communicators will also coordinate across sectors. They will anticipate how news and social media shape public perception and ensure that schools, public health agencies, and community leaders are amplifying a shared message. Tools like social listening (monitoring what questions are being asked in town halls, on social media, or in school inboxes) can help leaders adapt in real time. Trust, equity, and communication each matter on their own—but it is their combined power, in the real-time uncertainty of crisis, that makes the greatest difference. The chapters you have just read bring these principles to life through the stories of K–12 and public health leaders across the country. In this final section, we invite you to go one step further: to not just *remember* what worked, but to *embed* these principles into your day-to-day thinking and decision-making.

To take these commitments forward, reimagine the role of schools—not just as educational institutions, but as vital partners in public health. That reimagining begins with a mindset shift—one that acknowledges the broader role schools play in promoting safety, stability, and wellness for students, families, and entire communities.

▶ TAKING ON A PUBLIC HEALTH MINDSET

Before the pandemic, many of us saw public schools as ever-present, open-door fixtures. Year after year, generation after generation, schools enrolled cohorts of kindergarteners and launched young adults into post-secondary plans. When school bells stopped ringing in March 2020, we experienced firsthand just how central schools are. It became clear that schools do much more than educate—they offer safe, stable, and nurturing environments; foster social and emotional growth; and connect students with peers, role models, and trusted adults. Schools offer community within communities, serving as sites for social support networks, hot meals, health centers, and recreational programs. During the pandemic, it was also clear that students, staff, and families fared better when their schools and districts partnered with local public health agencies to deliver core public health functions.

K-12 leaders who created these types of school communities adopted a public health mindset. This does not mean that they became public health experts, but that they considered how district policies could advance public health within their schools and communities. This mindset laid the groundwork for developing partnerships with local public health agencies and community organizations that focused on protecting and improving the health of students, staff, families, and the broader community.

REFLECTIONS FROM THE FIELD: ADDRESSING UNCERTAINTY

John Zurbuchen, assistant superintendent at Davis School District in Utah, reflected on the challenges of having to make decisions with insufficient data during the pandemic, illustrating a public health mindset aimed at keeping students and staff safe.

> COVID-19 has proven the adage 'hindsight is twenty-twenty.' Certainly, if we knew what we know now, we would have adjusted some of our directives and responses. Yet, admitting that we'd change things in hindsight does not equate to 'we were incorrect' in our responses in the moment. The beauty and strength of science is that it constantly reexamines assumptions based on new information and data. Correctly, health and safety were paramount considerations in our initial actions and assumptions. We acted on the adage, 'Do the least harm.' If we were going to be wrong in our protocols, then we were going to err on the side of caution and safety for students and staff. Our protocols were based on the best science at the time.

When K-12 leaders adopt a public health mindset and build partnerships that have a shared commitment to trust, equity, and communication, they help schools and public health agencies work better together in the face of disruption. After natural disasters, school shootings, teacher strikes, or a global pandemic, it is K-12 leaders who must determine when and how to reopen buildings and what kinds of supports their communities will need to heal and move forward (Smith & Riley, 2012; Virella, 2022). K-12 leaders who adopt a public health mindset are better equipped to make these decisions because they have already built trusting relationships, established shared goals around equity, and created communication channels with their school stakeholders and local public health partners that can be activated when the next crisis emerges.

▶ EMPLOYING DIFFERENT PRACTICES IN DIFFERENT CONTEXTS

Perhaps unsurprisingly for a nation of nearly 350 million people, no method for navigating a public health crisis will work in every locale. Crisis response efforts need to address immediate needs while accounting for specific local context. Local variations in response will often be driven by the capacity of existing health services in the community, access to real-time funding, private sector partnerships, K-12 leadership priorities, state guidance, and community willingness or hesitancy.

From an equity perspective, districts with greater financial resources will be better positioned than under-resourced districts to contract with the private sector to support crisis response and recovery. Dr. Jill Bohnenkamp, associate professor at the University of Maryland's National Center for School Mental Health recalled, "School communities that already had robust health and mental health infrastructures were able to adapt their systems more quickly to meet the changing needs and circumstances of the COVID-19 pandemic." These districts are better positioned to pivot during a crisis. Those with fewer resources will likely struggle, again, to get very basic resources like soap for bathroom dispensers. For leaders in remote areas, urban districts, and underfunded jurisdictions, partnerships can offer access to expertise, material resources, and personnel support that can be especially critical for districts with fewer resources, districts that are geographically isolated, and districts that struggle with staffing shortages.

▶ MOVING FORWARD: CONTINUE TO BUILD PARTNERSHIPS

Building on what we've learned, we conclude with recommendations for strengthening partnerships—guidance for K–12 and public health leaders, and for all who are committed to keeping students learning during a crisis. The pandemic revealed the incredible potential that emerges when K-12 and public health systems work together, and it is important to continue to work together. In the early days of COVID-19, school and public health leaders had to make fast, high-stakes decisions with limited information. They learned to lean on one another—not just out of necessity, but out of shared responsibility.

That urgency built partnerships. It is important to continue these partnerships as the crisis fades from view. Commitments to trust, equity, and communication must become embedded in how K-12 and public health leaders engage with one another, how they design systems, and how they make decisions with communities. Maintaining this work means investing in relationships before the next emergency.

Create Regular Touchpoints

For those who want to build or strengthen cross-sector networks, intentionality matters. Instead of thinking about frequency of interactions or number of connections, leaders can consider which types of interactions and connections are most useful (Varda et al., 2008). In other words, leaders should focus on high-impact partnerships that bring distinct resources, perspectives, or expertise. Leaders might create regular points of connection between districts, public health departments, and community organizations, ideally within existing structures. Public health boards, for example, can reserve a seat for a district leader; school districts can invite public health officials to join their emergency planning teams.

This kind of intention matters just as much when public health practitioners deliver school-based programming—on topics like chronic disease prevention, healthy relationships, or opioid overdose prevention. In those moments, we encourage public health leaders not to treat schools simply as sites of delivery, but as full partners in the work, and we encourage K-12 leaders to think about how these topics align with work already underway in the district. Both K-12 and public health leaders alike benefit from considering what it means to coalesce around a shared mission and to engage in discussion about what they are learning from and with each other.

Share Data with Each Other

Using and sharing data are regular practices in successful partnerships. They help to build trust and support decision-making that is grounded in equity. Data help leaders see which groups need more resources and allows partners to make decisions that are fair and responsive. To ensure that partners can learn from each other's data before the next crisis, K-12 and public health leaders can develop HIPAA- and FERPA-compliant data-sharing agreements and develop information-sharing systems so that each has access to relevant data around specific areas of concern. For example, if public health leaders had data showing a sudden drop in school attendance during the flu season, they may work with the superintendent to develop a flu shot campaign or to host school-based flu shot events. When these data systems are developed prior to a public health crisis, leaders are able to efficiently act on the data when a crisis hits, instead of spending time developing systems to collect or share data.

Collaborate Around Emergency Planning

It is common for districts and public health agencies to engage in emergency planning, but this work is often done independently.

K-12 and public health leaders can make dedicated time to engage in emergency planning together. They can conduct role play planning exercises (see Appendix B), develop after-action reports to document lessons and strengthen future response, or participate in drills to practice coordinated responses. This type of planning requires ongoing communication between partners, and that communication also gives them time and space to learn more about the skills, expertise, resources, and services that each individual partner, and their respective organization, bring to bear. As this knowledge deepens, their capacity to respond increases: they know who to reach out to in a crisis and what partners can, and cannot provide.

▶ FINAL THOUGHTS

Natural disasters, disease outbreaks, and civil unrest create periods of uncertainty and challenge that require effective leadership and partnership. While the future is uncertain, during the pandemic we learned that resilience does not come from certainty—it comes from alignment. When public health and education leaders align their values, share their knowledge, and coordinate their actions, they can move more effectively, equitably, and confidently—even when the path ahead is unclear.

The work ahead will not be easy—but we are not starting from scratch. The partnerships formed during the pandemic, the hard-earned lessons, and the framework forged in real time give us a foundation to build from. We hope the stories of partnership, and the principles of trust, equity, and communication that they illustrate, will not remain distant ideals, but that readers take steps now to build and strengthen partnerships with their colleagues in K-12 and public health. That work will ensure that when the next crisis comes - and it will - schools and public health systems are ready to keep students safe, supported and learning.

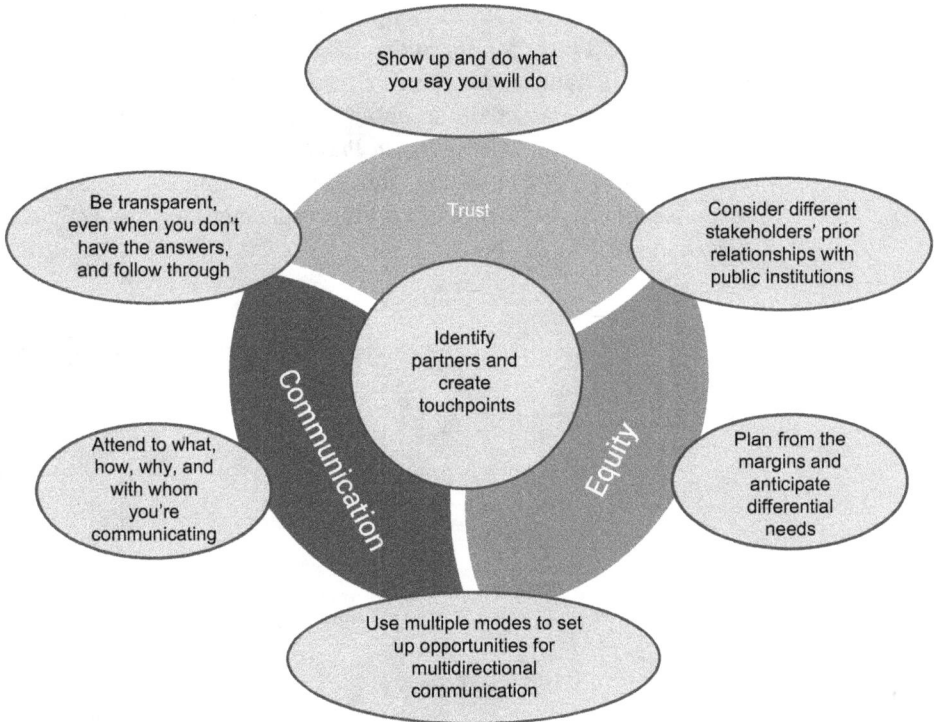

Figure 5.1 Partnership Framework: A Shared Commitment to Trust, Equity, and Effective Communication.

References

Leslie, J. (2023). *The Crisis of Trust in Public Health: Sociopolitical trends influence people's confidence in public health institutions.* Think Global Health. Retrieved from https://www.thinkglobalhealth. org/article/crisis-trust-public-health

Merod, A. (2022). *Nearly half of voters say trust in public education declined since pandemic.* Informa. Retrieved from https://www. k12dive.com/news/pandemic-declined-trust-public-education/ 637383/

Smith, L., & Riley, D. (2012). School leadership in times of crisis. *School Leadership & Management, 32*(1), 57–71.

Varda, D. M., Chandra, A., Stern, S. A., & Lurie, N. (2008). Core dimensions of connectivity in public health collaboratives. *Journal of Public Health Management and Practice, 14*(5), E1–E7.

Virella, P. M. (2022). Leading through the "influx:" Leadership responses and the influence of a political spectacle. *Journal of School Leadership, 32*(1), 27–50.

Afterword

When Leah Perkinson and her co-authors invited me to write the afterword for this book, I was honored—and a little daunted. How do you find words for what we've lived through, what we've learned, and what we're still carrying forward?

For context: I'm a pediatrician who transitioned from private practice to state public health in 2016. I became medical director of the Tennessee Department of Health's Vaccine-Preventable Diseases and Immunizations Program in January 2019. I walked into that role in the middle of a multi-state hepatitis A outbreak, which was soon followed by a measles outbreak. And then came reported deaths from a new respiratory virus in Wuhan, China.

In February 2020, I hosted a dinner party at our house. One guest asked, "What do you think of this new virus in China?" I said, "I think it's going to change every aspect of our lives." He laughed and dismissed it. His wife leaned in and said, "You *do* know what she does for a living, right?"

On March 5, Tennessee confirmed its first COVID-19 case— in my home county. My husband, a local school board member, and I were both immediately pulled into the response. While I fielded calls from hospitals, physicians, and local health departments, he tried to help the district navigate emerging risks. Within hours, schools closed. The assumption was they would reopen in a week or two. But when you close schools before there's a single case in the building, how do you justify reopening them again?

From that moment on, we were running at full speed. My staff tripled overnight. People talk about building the plane while flying it—ours was also on fire. Spring was a blur of case identification, contact tracing, drive-through high school graduations, and trying to understand the virus. By the summer of 2020, I was drafting reopening guidance for schools. And by fall, I was spending hours each week on statewide calls with superintendents. These weren't just technical briefings—they were lifelines. We created space to ask hard questions, share updates in real time, and learn alongside each other. Public health leaders didn't just answer questions—we worked beside leaders in education, translating policy into practice, strategy into logistics, and trying to anticipate what was coming next.

When the long-awaited vaccines became available in December 2020, we were ready. We wrote a plan for Tennessee's vaccine roll-out that was lauded as the most equitable and science-based plan in the nation. We vaccinated at a rate that outpaced nearly every other state. One of the best moments of the pandemic for me was when I had the honor of vaccinating a 95-year-old World War II veteran. We both cried.

But public enthusiasm didn't last, and demand waned. Rumors, conspiracy theories, and misleading health-related information surged.

And that's why those early meetings with superintendents mattered—and why the partnership that followed mattered even more. They revealed what the pandemic made impossible to ignore: public health and education are not just adjacent systems, but deeply interdependent. Our missions converge in every classroom and every community. And our ability to respond to today's public health challenges—and those still ahead—depends on how we work together, every step of the way.

And that's why this book matters. Because it offers more than a retrospective—it offers a framework built from hard-won lessons and a vision rooted in partnership. It reminds us that collaboration between K–12 and public health leaders isn't something we reserve for crises. It's something we invest in all the time.

To sustain that connection and coordination, we can approach our work and partnerships in ways that are grounded in trust, shaped by equity, and strengthened through effective communication. So what can we do—today—to begin?

We can start by reflecting not just on whether we show up, but *how* **we show up**. We can admit what we don't yet know and commit to digging until we find the answers. We can show up with empathy and extend understanding when tensions run high and professional facades start to crack. Because behind every title and role is a person doing their best.

We can also think carefully about what we bring. Sometimes it's technical support—walking through a confusing policy one on one or sending that simple, steady text message: "Working on it. We'll have an answer by the end of the week." Sometimes it's the willingness to make just one thing easier. And sometimes, it's the courage to take a data-informed risk—without a perfect blueprint, but with enough evidence to try something that might make things better for kids. We act not because we're certain, but because we're committed.

Where disparities are ignored, trust will falter. Together, K–12 and public health leaders can commit to working toward equitable outcomes, through equitable processes. We can analyze data by race and language, and ask and answer hard questions like: **Who is being left behind?** and, **Who will and will not benefit from this program?** We can focus on students who face the greatest barriers, and prioritize resources based on need. We can tailor strategies so they're accessible and acceptable— shaped by culture, language, and lived experience. And we can ask families and students what trust looks like to them and ask them about the people in their communities who carry credibility.

This is the work of equity. It is intentional, ongoing, and shared. And it's how we build systems that are worthy of the trust we seek.

Today, we can apply principles of effective communication— because communication is the throughline that connects everything else. It's how trust is built and how equity is made visible. We can communicate clearly, consistently, and with care, and in doing so, create the conditions for people to feel heard, respected, and included. We can develop proactive plans that are shared across sectors, that center community voice from the beginning, trade jargon for clarity, and adapt core messages so they resonate with the intended audiences. And we can encourage educators to help shape public health messages—and public health professionals to co-design what success looks like in schools.

And the truth is, we don't have to do all of this at once. Just one small shift—one conversation, one change in approach—can help move us forward. Because we need to shift the trajectory. We need to build the systems that will carry us through today's challenges and whatever comes next. And we need to do it now—because we are already in a time that demands more of us than ever before.

It doesn't have to be perfect. But it does have to be purposeful. And it has to be right. And being right sometimes means saying, "we don't know yet," and helping everyone understand that we're making the best possible recommendations given the information we have at the time. That information will change and, when it does, so will those guidelines.

Today feels like the ground is still shifting under our feet—politically, socially, culturally. The pressure on public health and education is relentless, and the stakes are high. But even in uncertainty, we have choices. We can let go of what we can't control and focus our energy on where we can make a difference. When we do that—when we work together with urgency and humility—we turn hard times into meaningful progress.

Earlier this year, I was invited to speak to pediatric residents at West Virginia University about advocacy. Honestly, I struggled to prepare. How do you talk about advocacy with young physicians who are overwhelmed and watching systems unravel in front of them? Then, just days before the talk, my 85-year-old mom fell and broke her hip. I flew back to Tennessee to help her recover. Sitting in her hospital room as she slept, I thought about everything she's seen since 1939: World War II, the Holocaust, the Cuban Missile Crisis, the moon landing, the Vietnam War, home computers, cell phones, social media, COVID-19...

And I thought: in the arc of a life, this moment we're in? It's a blip.

One of my favorite children's books is *Alexander and the Terrible, Horrible, No Good, Very Bad Day* by Judith Viorst. For that talk, I took a screenshot of the cover, crossed out the word "Day," and replaced it with "BLIP." The Terrible, Horrible, No Good, Very Bad... *Blip.*

And that's what I told the residents. Yes, we're in a hard season. But it's just that—a season. And like every season, it will pass.

In the meantime, yes, we should be doing everything we can to lessen the height and duration of this blip. But we should also be making sure that when we get to the other side, we've done the work—together—to build something better.

That's what this book offers: not a conclusion, but a beginning. A framework to move forward. A reminder that partnership isn't a one-time fix—it's an ongoing relationship. We don't need to have all the answers. But we do need to commit. One act of follow-through. One coordinated message. One risk worth taking. These are the choices that build better systems—stronger, more connected, and more prepared leaders. We WILL get there, together.

See you on the other side.

Michelle Fiscus, MD, FAAP
Chief Medical Officer, Association
of Immunization Managers (AIM)

Support Material

The appendices in this book are also available on the book product page online, so you can easily print them for use. To access these downloads, go to www.routledge.com/9781041002383 and click on the "Support Material" link.

- Appendix B
- Appendix C
- Appendix E
- Appendix F

Appendix A: Contributing Participant Biographies

▶ **Mara G. Aspinall, MBA**, Partner, Illumina Ventures and Former Advisor to The Rockefeller Foundation

For Mara Aspinall, a typical day in her role includes evaluating up-and-coming diagnostic technologies, working with existing companies to expand and promote testing, and teaching biomedical diagnostics at Arizona State University. During the pandemic, Mara's main focus was supporting programs and initiatives that advocate for regular COVID testing – particularly in K-12 schools. Mara drew upon her 35+ year background in the areas of diagnostics, genomics, and personalized medicine to become a national authority and advocate for COVID testing. When Mara is not working, she enjoys hiking with friends, adding to her extensive Oreo cookie collection, and cheering on the Boston Red Sox.

▶ **Leslie Bergstrom, EdD**, Oregon School District Superintendent, Oregon, Wisconsin

Dr. Leslie Bergstrom is the Superintendent of Schools for the Oregon School District (OSD) in Wisconsin, which is located just south of Madison and serves over 4,300 students in pre-kindergarten – grade 12. As a lifelong educator, Dr. Bergstrom has had the opportunity to lead in a wide variety of capacities in public schools, including classroom teaching, curriculum design, and administration. Her career is marked by dedication to students and families, collaborative leadership, and a focus on educational equity. Under her leadership, OSD has become known for fostering an environment where students thrive academically, socially, and emotionally.

▶ **Jill Bohnenkamp, PhD**, Associate Professor, National Center for School Mental Health, Division of Child and Adolescent Psychiatry, University of Maryland School of Medicine, Baltimore, Maryland

Dr. Bohnenkamp is an associate professor and core faculty at the National Center for School Mental Health at the University of Maryland School of Medicine and a licensed clinical psychologist. For Jill, a typical day includes consultation and technical assistance to school, district, and state mental health and education leaders across the United States to help them advance and sustain comprehensive school mental health systems in their communities. During the pandemic, Dr. Bohnenkamp supported school, district, and state leaders as they responded to the increasing prevalence and severity of children's mental health needs and shifted service models to respond to changing school environments. When Jill is not working, she enjoys watching her daughters play soccer and spending time outside.

▶ **Diana Bruce**, Founder and CEO, Diana Bruce and Associates LLC

Diana Bruce, CEO and Founder of Diana Bruce and Associates LLC, brings 25+ years experience in health and education policy, working across government, schools, health care providers, and nonprofits. Diana provides strategic planning, stakeholder engagement, policy development, and training and coaching, delivering empathy-based, policy-driven, human-centered solutions to her clients and their constituents. During the COVID-19 pandemic, Diana supported K-12 schools with disease mitigation and testing strategies, and led nationwide communities of practice on implementing testing programs in schools. Diana often serves on nonprofit boards and holds a Master of Public Administration and Policy from Columbia University.

▶ **Sheretta Butler-Barnes, PhD**, Professor, Washington University, Brown School of Social Work, St. Louis, Missouri

Dr. Sheretta Butler-Barnes is a professor at the WashU Brown School of Social Work, with affiliations in African and African American studies and data and computational sciences. A developmental psychologist, her research examines how racism and cultural strengths impact the health and wellbeing of Black American families. In 2023–24, she served as the Inaugural Sojourner Truth Visiting Professor at Rutgers University. She holds a PhD and MA from Wayne State University and a BS from Michigan State. Her research includes the Black Families and Racial Justice Project and the Equity for Black Women and Girls Project.

▶   **Andrea L. Cahn**, Senior Vice President of Special Olympics Unified Champion Schools, Special Olympics North America

Andrea has been with Special Olympics for 36 years and has held a variety of leadership roles in communications, program strategy development, and government relations. She draws on all of her experience in her current position, responsible for a $36 million per year partnership with the US Department of Education that promotes social inclusion by creating model schools of acceptance through the innovative implementation of Special Olympics Unified Sports, inclusive youth leadership, and other school wide education and awareness activities. Andrea oversees implementation strategy, research, and evaluation for Unified Champion Schools programming in nearly 11,00 schools, providing more than 18 million inclusive experiences to students across the country each year.

During and since the pandemic, Andrea's emphasis has been on ensuring that the resources and activities made available to Unified Champion Schools educators were converted to virtual and hybrid modalities and providing the additional professional development and teacher supports needed for success. Ensuring that students with ID/IDD, already at risk for isolation, disengagement, and exclusion, were not further isolated during the pandemic has been a major challenge.

Andrea found her passion for inclusion as a volunteer with children with intellectual disabilities beginning in 1968. She holds a degree in special education and language development and has taught second and fourth grades in Appalachian Virginia. She currently resides in Alexandria, Virginia.

▶   **Hannah Carter**, Project Manager, School District Environmental Health, Center for Green Schools at the US Green Building Council, St Louis, Missouri

Hannah Carter supports school district staff working to improve air quality by coordinating education and training through the Center's School Air Quality Leaders Network. Prior to joining the Center for Green Schools in early 2022, Hannah was the sustainability coordinator at Parkway School District and led initiatives to improve indoor air quality district-wide and support the district's pandemic response. When Hannah's not working, she enjoys hiking and attempting home renovation projects.

▶ **Saurabh Chandra, MD, PhD**, Chief Telehealth Officer, University of Mississippi Medical Center, Center for Telehealth/ Telehealth Center of Excellence

Dr. Chandra is the chief telehealth officer at University of Mississippi Medical Center (UMMC) and project director for the National Center of Excellence for Telehealth. The Center for Telehealth at UMMC is one of the only two federally designated Centers of Excellence for Telehealth in the country. In his current role, Dr. Chandra provides strategic direction to the Center for Telehealth and ensures alignment with all three mission areas of UMMC.

▶ **Brittany Choate, MSC**, Director of Programs, Saliva-Direct, Yale University School of Public Health, New Haven, Connecticut

Brittany is an accomplished program director and stakeholder engagement specialist. She leverages her expertise to build and manage innovative solutions that address complex social challenges – from water conservation programming to an Emmy® Award–winning documentary to first-of-its-kind outbreak response models. Brittany has a proven record of building community-driven programs, utilizing her skills in developing strategic partnerships, driving equity and inclusion initiatives, and partnering with diverse communities to take meaningful action. Currently, Brittany serves as Director of Programs for the public health nonprofit SalivaDirect, Inc., where she oversees an expanding portfolio of initiatives that aim to increase health equity and access in traditionally underserved communities.

▶ **Rhiannon Clifton, BS, MBA**, Senior Director, Office of Strategic Initiatives, University of Illinois System and Former Senior Director of Integration, SHIELD Illinois

Rhiannon Clifton served as Senior Director of Integration at SHIELD Illinois, a statewide COVID-19 testing initiative deploying the University of Illinois' innovative saliva test. From 2021 to 2023, she led testing operations, customer success, and labs, supporting over 7 million tests across 1,700 partner sites, including schools, universities, businesses, and community organizations. In this chief operations role, she built integrated operations, developed talent, and helped guide the organization through rapid scale-up and wind-down phases. Her work ensured accessible, reliable COVID-19 testing for Illinois residents during a time of urgent public need. Rhiannon holds a BS in advertising and an MBA.

▶ **Elizabeth Coke, MEd**, Acting Deputy, Emergency Preparedness and Response Branch, Centers for Disease Control and Prevention

Elizabeth Coke possesses extensive expertise in managing complex projects, strategic planning, resource optimization, and partnership development. With more than 30 years of experience in adolescent and school health, she joined the CDC in 2005 after her tenure at the Michigan Department of Education, where she implemented CDC's chronic disease and HIV prevention programs. During the pandemic, Eliz coordinated operations for the School Support Section of CDC's COVID-19 Response. As an educator, protecting the students and staff in all education settings has been her priority. Outside of work, Elizabeth enjoys spending time with her adult children and friends, gardening, reading, and relaxing by the water.

▶ **Ann Covey, MSN, RN, NCSN**, Education Associate, School Health Services and State School Nurse Consultant, Delaware Department of Education

Ann Covey serves as the education associate for School Health Services at the Delaware Department of Education and is Delaware's State School Nurse Consultant. She supports the School Nurse Certification Program, monitors compliance and data, provides professional development, offers technical assistance, and facilitates a statewide Community of Practice for school nurses. Ann brings over 14 years of school nursing experience and a decade as a pediatric emergency/trauma nurse to her role. Outside of work, Ann enjoys family dinners, game nights, boating, snow tubing, and beach trips with her husband, their five amazing daughters, and her two sons-in-law.

▶ **Deborah D'Souza-Vazirani DrPH, MHSA**, Director, Program Evaluation, Grants, and External Partners, National Association of School Nurses

Dr. D'Souza-Vazirani is a public health specialist responsible for program evaluation at the National Association of School Nurses (NASN). She managed NASN's Champions for School Health initiative which focused on increasing pediatric vaccine access, confidence, and uptake. She worked to engage school nurses and community-based organizations to develop innovative programming in vaccine confidence and equity. Her background is in health equity research and evaluation with a focus on child health delivery systems.

▶ **Jason Dropik**, School Administrator, Indian Community School, and Board Member/Parliamentarian, National Indian Education Association

Mr. Dropik previously served as the school administrator for the Indian Community School supporting students in building a strong Native Identity and preparing for continued success. His current role is Executive Director for the National Indian Education Association. During the pandemic, Mr. Dropik was focused on ensuring that students and staff had a safe space to learn and grow together. His experience in building community and innovative solutions helped to successfully keep his school open throughout the pandemic (except when prohibited by the state). When Mr. Dropik is not working, he enjoys continued learning, serving various communities, and spending time with his family, especially outdoors.

▶ **Heather M. Drummond, MPH**, Senior Director, Health Systems and Workforce Transformation and Former Testing Branch Manager, COVID-19 Response, Washington State Department of Health

Heather Drummond serves as Senior Director, Health Systems and Workforce Transformation at the Washington State Department of Health, overseeing the agency's rural health, primary care, health workforce, and healthcare engagement efforts. Heather previously served as COVID-19 Vaccine Director and COVID-19 Testing Manager, supporting the Learn to Return school testing program and Say Yes! COVID Test. Heather's previous work experience includes supporting YMCAs to formally connect with healthcare, health system strengthening efforts domestically and internationally, and local health department capacity building. Heather holds a master's degree in public health from the University of Illinois at Chicago, and a bachelor's degree from the University of Washington.

▶ **John Eisenberg**, Executive Director, National Association of State Directors of Special Education, Alexandria, Virginia

On December 4, 2018, John Eisenberg assumed the role of Executive Director of the National Association of State Directors of Special Education (NASDSE). Before this new role, Mr. Eisenberg worked in the Office of Special Education and Student Services at the Virginia Department of Education for fifteen years, seven of those as the State Director of Special Education. Throughout his career in special education, he worked in a variety of other roles including director of the Virginia Deaf-Blind Project, technical assistance specialist with the National Technical Assistance Consortium for Deaf-Blindness, and a classroom teacher for students with developmental disabilities and Deaf-Blindness. He comes from a family of teachers and special educators and is very passionate about improving the educational outcomes of children and families across the United States.

▶ **Mary Ellen Engel, MSN, RN, NJ-CSN**, Nursing Supervisor (retired), North Brunswick Township Schools, New Jersey

For Mary Ellen, a typical day in her role included collaborating with the nursing staff, interdisciplinary teams, and district leaders to develop appropriate health care plans and policies to ensure students are safe, healthy, and ready to learn in school.

During the pandemic, Mary Ellen's main focus was developing district-wide plans to mitigate the spread of COVID-19, to utilize technology to capture, analyze, and disseminate accurate data, and to provide accessible resources and services to the school community. Mary Ellen recently retired from her position as district nursing supervisor for North Brunswick Township School District and is thoroughly enjoying spending time with her six grandchildren and volunteering in her community.

▶ **Meagan Fitzpatrick, PhD**, Assistant Professor, Center for Vaccine Development and Global Health, University of Maryland School of Medicine, Baltimore, Maryland

Dr. Fitzpatrick is an infectious disease transmission modeler, a job description not particularly well known prior to COVID-19. During the pandemic, Meagan's main focus was evaluating mitigation policies for K-12 educational settings. Meagan drew on her background modeling other respiratory infections such as influenza, RSV, and pertussis to do this work, as well as emerging pathogens such as Zika. She also drew upon her experience as a parent to two boys and her community of parents and educators, who frequently raised important questions. When Meagan's not working, she likes to garden, travel with her family, and tell corny jokes.

▶ **Emily Frank, MD, FAAP**, Associate Professor of Pediatrics, University of California San Francisco, Director of Health Education Partnerships: Oakland, Health Teacher, Life Academy, AAP Council on School Health Executive Committee, Oakland, California

Dr. Emily Frank is an associate professor of pediatrics at the University of California, San Francisco. She is a board-certified pediatrician who practices in the Teen Clinics and School-Based Health Centers at Benioff Children's Hospital Oakland and a public school teacher in the Oakland Unified School District. During the early pandemic, her daily work involved taking care of children with suspected COVID in the emergency rooms and primary care clinics, remote and hybrid classroom teaching, and supporting the Oakland Unified School District in planning for a safe transition to in-person learning.

▶ **Julia Daisy Fraustino, PhD**, Associate Professor of Strategic Communication and Director of the Public Interest Communication Research Laboratory at West Virginia University in Morgantown

Julia is an award-winning risk, crisis, and disaster communication scientist and strategic communication educator. She works to enhance resilience to risk and disasters through leveraging the power of communities and strong communication that is informed by rigorous social and behavioral science. During a typical day in her roles, in addition to teaching and mentoring students in the classroom and in the lab, she also leads multiple public interest research projects with state and national partners focusing on data-driven strategic communication that helps people move their minds, hearts, and actions for the better for themselves and society. During the COVID-19 pandemic Julia led the Joint Information Center, the coordinated, evidence-based, community-engaged communication arm of the state of West Virginia's pandemic response.

▶ **Stefanie Friedhoff**, Associate Professor of the Practice of Health Services, Policy and Practice, Co-Founder of the Information Futures Lab, Brown University School of Public Health, Providence, R.I.

Stefanie Friedhoff is co-founder of the Information Futures Lab; lead investigator of the STAT Network, a peer network of over 600 state public health leaders responding to infectious disease and other public health challenges; and Professor of the Practice at the Brown University School of Public Health. An expert in media, communications, and global health strategy, she focuses on information ecosystems and health equity. From July 2022 to May 2023, Friedhoff served as a senior policy advisor on the White House COVID-19 Response Team, focusing on population information needs, health equity, community engagement, and medical countermeasure uptake. Previously, she held leadership roles at the Harvard Global Health Institute and The Nieman Foundation for Journalism at Harvard, creating programs on trauma journalism and global health reporting. The former journalist's work has appeared in *TIME*, *The Boston Globe*, and international publications.

▶ **María Virginia Giani, M. Ed.**, Graduate student, University of Florida and Former Curriculum and Behavior Specialist with Alachua County Public Schools, Florida

At the beginning of the pandemic, María Virginia virtually taught her students and then, a few months into the pandemic, transitioned to a district role where she supported professionals with learning how to teach in virtual and hyflex settings while continuing to support students, families, and schools with curriculum and behavior. In August of 2022, María Virginia began her PhD studies at the University of Florida, under Project EASE: Econometric Analysis of Special Education. She hopes to continue to advocate for students with disabilities and center their voices and experiences while helping create more equitable educational spaces.

▶ **Jenna Grant**, Grant Specialist, Ascension St. John and Former Resource Development Manager, Tulsa Health Department, Oklahoma

As the former resource development manager for Tulsa Health Department and its nonprofit branch, Pathways to Health, Jenna brought useful services when and where they were most needed. She was a proud member of the Cross-City Learning Group during the COVID pandemic, helping the largest public school district in Tulsa reopen to in-person instruction and implementing trauma-informed training in local schools and agencies.

▶ **Emily E. Haroz, PhD, MHS, MA**, Associate Professor, Johns Hopkins Center for Indigenous Health, Johns Hopkins Bloomberg School of Public Health, Baltimore, MD

Dr. Haroz joined the Center for Indigenous Health in July of 2016. She has extensive experience in the implementation and evaluation of programs addressing mental and behavioral health. Her background is in quantitative methods, advanced statistical approaches, and epidemiology. She has conducted numerous studies to understand mental and behavioral health problems and programs across a wide range of diverse populations. Dr. Haroz's current research leverages implementation science, machine learning, and mixed methods to address mental and behavioral health concerns and promote well-being among AI/

AN communities. Recent projects include *Family Spirit Strengths*, a home-visiting intervention supporting parents and caregivers experiencing mental distress and substance misuse (funded by NIDA), and *Reclaiming Indigenous Children's Futures Through Home-Visiting and Intergenerational Playspaces* (funded by the LEGO Foundation).

▶ **Jennifer Harper**, Consultant

Jennifer is a trailblazer who specializes in launching cross-sector initiatives, projects, and programs in partnerships in order to elevate the quality of life in her community. Jennifer has a proven record of collaborating on major campaigns that deliver success. As an accomplished professional leader and strategist, she has launched local, regional, and statewide initiatives to become sustained organizations and/or programs. Her success and results are complimented by a belief in nurturing those in her community. Jennifer has a master's degree in public administration from the University of Oklahoma and is a certified project management professional through PMI.

▶ **Dina Hasiotis McEvoy, MPA**, Chief Strategy Officer, Attuned Education Partners and Former Chief School Support and Improvement Officer, New Orleans Public Schools

For Dina, her typical day during the pandemic was helping public schools identify their greatest challenges and developing plans to better support students throughout their educational journeys. Dina's main focus was ensuring schools in New Orleans Public Schools were open, safe, and equitably providing resources and supports to students, with specific attention paid to distribution of technology in the spring of 2020, building a roadmap to safely open schools citywide in August of 2020, and organizing efforts to ensure all students and families had access to COVID-19 testing. Dina drew on her experience in convening leaders, building solutions and relationships, and implementing policies with school and city partners, along with her passion for educational equity, to do this work. When Dina's not working, she likes to entertain friends and spend time with her husband and two daughters, Zoe and Samantha, both students in New Orleans public schools.

▶ **Jeremiah Hay, MPP**, Associate Commissioner of Operations Strategy and Intelligence, Massachusetts Department of Transitional Assistance and Former Acting Chief of Staff, Massachusetts Executive Office of Health and Human Services

Jeremiah was born and raised in New York City and studied politics and history at Oberlin College before working on several political campaigns and then spending five years advocating for and then implementing Universal Pre-K in NYC. After completing an MPP at Harvard's Kennedy School, he joined Massachusetts' COVID-19 Command Center, where he led efforts on COVID testing and school reopening. Jeremiah held a number of roles at the Executive Office of Health and Human Services, including acting chief of staff. In September 2024, he joined the MA Department of Transitional Assistance as the Associate Commissioner of Operations Strategy and Intelligence.

▶ **Karen Heath**, Director of Communications, Berrien Regional Education Service Agency (RESA), Berrien Springs, Michigan and Vice President, National School Public Relations Association, Mideast Region

During the initial stages of the pandemic, Karen—along with her Michigan School Public Relations Association colleagues—developed a series of toolkits for school leaders to use to communicate what to "Do First" as students and families were processing abrupt school closures, what to do "Before Schools Open" when districts began to welcome students back, and what to do when "Schools Are Open and Operating" as schools dealt with positive cases, outbreaks, and potential future closures. During that time, she also helped develop Governor Gretchen Whitmer's communication plan to roll out the Disaster Relief Child Care Services for Michigan's Essential Workforce program and worked with the Berrien County Health Department to author a resource guide for families so that everyone had access to the same protocols and expectations relative to symptom screening, quarantine expectations, and isolation procedures.

▶ **Ashley Hill, MPH, MBA**, Associate Director, State and Territory Alliance for Testing, Brown University School of Public Health, Providence, Rhode Island

Since 2022, Ashley Hill has led the day-to-day operations of the STAT Network, a peer network of state health department leaders. Prior to STAT, she served as a state assistant administrator at the Michigan Department of Health and Human Services, playing a key role in Michigan's COVID-19 response—leading efforts in contact tracing, community testing, and establishing a FEMA mass vaccination site in Detroit. Before the pandemic, Ashley focused on behavioral and physical health integration for Michigan's Medicaid population, and on improving health policy from all angles (legislative, executive, public company, nonprofit, member association, foundation). She lives in Detroit with her family.

▶ **Greg Holzman, MD, MPH**, Holzman Consulting, and Former State Medical Officer with Montana Department of Public Health and Human Services, Helena, Montana

Dr. Greg Holzman is the former state medical officer for the Department of Public Health and Human Services. During the pandemic, Dr. Holzman was part of the governor's COVID-19 task force working with the team on the pandemic response. Greg is board certified in family medicine and preventive medicine and public health. He has worked in academia, research, clinical medicine, and state and federal public health.

▶ **Tracy Jentz, APR**, Director of Survey Research, Donovan Group and Former Communications and Community Engagement Coordinator, Grand Forks Public Schools, North Dakota; North Central Region Vice President, National School Public Relations Association,

Tracy Jentz, APR, is the director of survey research at the Donovan Group, a nationally renowned communications firm exclusively serving public education. Before joining the Donovan Group, Tracy spent more than 10 years as communications coordinator for one of the largest school systems in North Dakota, where she provided a strategic communications and research focus through her award-winning work. She has presented at several state and national school communications conferences and served a three-year term on the National School Public Relations Association (NSPRA) Executive Board.

▶ **Russell D. Johnston, PhD**, Superintendent, Wallingford-Swarthmore School District, Wallingford, Pennsylvania and Former Acting Commissioner, Massachusetts Department of Elementary and Secondary Education

Dr. Russell D. Johnston is the superintendent of the Wallingford-Swarthmore School District. With a lifelong passion for education and a deep commitment to student success, Dr. Johnston has a wealth of experience in leadership, special education, and instructional support. Johnston was most recently acting commissioner of elementary and secondary education in Massachusetts where he worked closely with schools and communities to enhance learning opportunities for all students. Throughout his career, he has been dedicated to fostering inclusive, supportive, and high-achieving school environments. His leadership has focused on empowering educators, strengthening student services, and building collaborative partnerships with families and the community. Before stepping into state-level leadership, Dr. Johnston was the superintendent of West Springfield Public Schools and has also served as a special education director and an inclusion facilitator.

▶ **Cathy Kedjidjian, APR**, Current Chief Communications Officer, Deerfield Public Schools District 109, Deerfield, Illinois and Former Executive Director of Communications & Strategic Planning, Glenview School District 34, Glenview, Illinois, Former President, National School Public Relations Association

For Cathy Kedjidjian, APR, a typical day in school communications is never predictable, but always focuses on strategically and personally creating clarity and connections. During the pandemic, a primary focus for Cathy was ensuring that staff had information first, and the tools and skills to communicate with students and parents. Cathy drew on her background in political campaigns, healthcare communications, and on her care and concern about the staff, students, and families who, more than ever, needed quick and easy access to information. When Cathy's not working, she runs, bikes, swims, meditates, and eats a lot of kale.

▶ **Marlee (Kingsley) Carlos**, Founder & CEO, JourneyUp Solutions, LLC and Former Principal with Rios Partners, Arlington, Virginia

For Marlee (Kingsley) Carlos, a typical day in her role includes helping nonprofits, their boards, and their leaders be more effective at achieving results, advising clients on strategic planning, and coaching leaders. During the pandemic, Marlee's main focus was on working with nonprofit clients to develop and launch strategies in the education, immigration, and anti-human trafficking space. Marlee drew on her background as a teacher to do this work. When Marlee's not working, she likes to hike and host cooking gatherings with her friends and neighbors.

▶ **Jessica Kjar**, Compliance Specialist, CITTA Brokerage Company (CBC) and Former COVID-19 K-12 School Testing Program Manager, Office of Emerging Infections, Utah Department of Health and Human Services

During the pandemic, Jessica spent four years focusing on managing K-12 testing needs for the State of Utah. Her work centered on administering CARES, CRSSA, ESSER, and ARP ESSER Funds at the Utah State School Board before transitioning to the Utah Department of Health and Human Services. Utilizing her background in politics and crisis management, she tackled pressing public health challenges during this critical time. Now, Jessica has shifted to the private sector while continuing to engage with compliance-related work. In her free time, she loves Harry Potter and supports the University of Tennessee (Go VOLS), while enjoying family time with her husband and 6-year-old son.

▶ **Brittany Layman, RN, BSN, NCSN**, Director of Health, Wellness and Safety, Regional School Unit 22, Hampden, Maine

For Brittany Layman, a typical day in her role includes verifying that health service staffing levels are appropriate, managing the district's comprehensive safety plan, and facilitating a Farm and Sea to School program. During the pandemic, Brittany's main focus was on implementing a robust testing program using pooled and antigen testing. Brittany drew on her background with school health and inpatient acute care to do this work. When Brittany's not working, she enjoys coaching and playing volleyball with her two daughters.

▶ **Sonia Lee, PhD**, Branch Chief, Maternal and Pediatric Infectious Disease Branch, Eunice Kennedy Shriver National Institute of Child Health and Human Development (NICHD)-National Institutes of Health

For Sonia Lee, a typical day in her role includes collaborating with research investigators on pediatric and adolescent infectious disease prevention and treatment. During the pandemic, Sonia's main focus was on the NIH RADx-UP Safe Return to School Diagnostic Testing Initiative to address the needs of underserved and vulnerable populations in their safe return to in-person learning. Sonia drew on her background and experience with behavioral science and HIV-AIDS to do this work. When Sonia's not working, she likes to spend time with her loved ones outdoors.

▶ **Kathy León, BS, RN, NCSN**, Lead District Nurse, San Gabriel Unified School District, San Gabriel, California

For Kathy, a typical day in her role includes direct student care, care coordination, special education assessments, mandated screenings, health education, and lots of meetings. During the pandemic, Kathy's main focus was on meeting the physical and mental health needs of her school community while continuing to attend to the "typical" school nurse duties. Kathy drew on her background in school health and experience working with students, staff, and families to do this work. When Kathy's not working, she likes to read, watch sports, and coach multiple sports with Special Olympics.

▶ **Jennifer Lepard, DrPH, MPA**, Partner at Lepard Group and Former Chief of Health, Wellness and Community Partnerships, Oklahoma State Department of Education, Oklahoma City, Oklahoma

For Jennifer, a typical day in her role during the pandemic included consulting with Oklahoma's 540+ school districts and her colleagues at the Oklahoma State Department of Health. During the pandemic, Jennifer worked at the State Department of Health, where she learned firsthand the important role school districts play in garnering community buy-in for public health initiatives. This inspired Jennifer to work with school districts full time through her role at the State Department of Education, focused on building long-term infrastructure to support and promote community health. When Jennifer's not working as an Oklahoma lobbyist at the Lepard Group, she likes to do puzzles, a hobby she took up long before it became popular in lockdown.

▶ **Robert Machak, EdD**, Superintendent of Schools, Woodland CCSD 50, Gurnee, Illinois

Dr. Robert Machak has served Woodland as superintendent for the past three years. His daily responsibilities include checking in with Woodland's four principals and seven program directors, and visiting at least one of the district's schools in person. During the pandemic, Dr. Machak implemented mitigation strategies necessary to safely keep Woodland's schools open for its 5,000 students and 1,000 staff members. Dr. Machak drew upon his previous role as associate superintendent of education, where he acted as the district's safety and security officer to do this work. Dr. Machak and his family enjoy spending time outdoors together.

▶ **Eric Masten**, Director of Federal Affairs, Education, The American Speech-Language-Hearing Association (ASHA), Rockville, Maryland

As the American Speech-Language-Hearing Association's Director of Federal Affairs, Education, Eric is ASHA's lead advocate on education issues with Congress and the administration. During the COVID-19 pandemic, this work focused on ensuring that school-based speech-language pathologists and educational audiologists — as well as other specialized instructional support personnel — had access to appropriate resources and administrative guidance to continue providing appropriate services while protecting the safety, health, and well-being of themselves, their families, and the students they serve. Eric has over 20 years of policy experience on Capitol Hill and with nonprofits at the national, state, and local levels, on a wide range of domestic policy issues. When not working, Eric enjoys running and exploring the mid-Atlantic with his husband.

▶ **Marnie (Margaret) McKercher DNP, MPH, RN, NCSN,** Lead School Nurse Consultant, Aurora Public Schools Health Services, Aurora, Colorado and University of Colorado College of Nursing Adjunct Clinical Faculty

Dr. McKercher is a school nurse administrator who collaborates with school nurses and district administration to provide health prevention initiatives and systems to remove health-related barriers for students with health needs. She was integral to the school district's pandemic response including partnerships with local and state public health departments, staff education, the development of district-wide COVID protocols and software, and implementation of school-located vaccination events. Her background is in the management of school nurses including hiring and professional development as well as the development of systems that address the needs of students with complex health needs.

▶ **Sheri McPartlin, MEd, BSN, RN,** Chief Nurse and Director of Employee and Student Health Services for the Clark County School District, Nevada

Sheri McPartlin is the Chief Nurse and Director of Employee and Student Health Services for the Clark County School District (CCSD), the fifth-largest school district in the United States, serving over 300,000 students and employing approximately 42,000 staff members across both urban and rural schools. In her role, Ms. McPartlin is responsible for the development and implementation of safe health policies and procedures across the district. She oversees the Health Services Department, which includes more than 260 school nurses, and provides expert consultation to CCSD administrators, as well as community and state agencies, on the administration of a comprehensive school health program. Her leadership was instrumental during the COVID-19 pandemic, as she guided CCSD through the crisis by pivoting to meet needs and challenges of the school community. With over 28 years of nursing experience, including expertise in both critical care and school health, Ms. McPartlin brings a wealth of knowledge and dedication to her work. She holds a Bachelor of Nursing from Oakland University, a Master of Education degree from Regis University, and an Educational Leadership Administrative Endorsement from Nova University.

▶ **Lynne P. Meadows, MS, BSN, RN, FNASN**, Director, District Health Services, Fulton County Schools, Georgia

For Lynne Meadows, a typical day in her role includes managing, directing, and supporting all school health staff, programs, and services. During the pandemic, Lynne's focus was helping to lead her district in their response, which included developing protocols and procedures, initiating safety mitigation strategies, providing education, interfacing with state, county, and other local health officials, oversight of all vaccination efforts, and school-located vaccination clinics. Lynne drew on her 30 years of nursing leadership, hospital, public health, and school nurse experience to do this work. When Lynne is not working, she likes to spend time with her family, travel, golf, and exercise. Lynne received an award from her school district and several other recognitions for her leadership during the pandemic.

▶ **Jeannine Foredich Medvedich**, Current Senior District and School Improvement Facilitator with WestEd and former Chief Academic Officer, Chief Leschi Schools, Tribal STEC School, Puyallup, Washington,

For Jeannine Medvedich, a typical day in her role includes serving as a district administrator, chief academic officer, in the superintendent's office, leading K-12 curriculum and instruction initiatives, professional development, intervention, special education, CTE, grant writing and oversight, and support of building administrators. This work includes long-term planning as well as daily problem solving around many logistics. During the pandemic, Jeannine's main focus was on making sure that students had access and received high quality uninterrupted instruction in a safe environment, ensuring that safety protocols were implemented. Jeannine drew on her background in/experience with over 25 years in education, having served as a building administrator at all grade levels to do this work, as well as being a mother of four during a major pandemic. When Jeannine's not working, she likes to get extra laundry done while spending time with her family.

▶ **Jason G. Newland MD, M.Ed.**, Division Chief of Pediatric Infectious Diseases at Nationwide Children's Hospital, Professor of Pediatrics and the Henry G Cramblett Chair in Medicine at The Ohio State University and Former Professor of Pediatrics, Pediatric Infectious Diseases, Vice Chair of Community Health and Strategic Planning, Washington University, St. Louis, MO

Dr. Jason Newland is the division chief of Pediatric Infectious Diseases at Nationwide Children's Hospital, a professor of pediatrics and the Henry G Cramblett Chair in Medicine at The Ohio State University. Prior to joining Nationwide Children's Hospital, he spent 10 years at Children's Mercy Hospital in Kansas City, MO and 8 years at Washington University School of Medicine in St. Louis. During the COVID-19 pandemic, Jason led ommunity-based research efforts evaluating the rate of transmission in schools, the impact of routine school-based SARS-CoV-2 testing, and effectiveness and safety of COVID-19 vaccines for children.

▶ **Brandi O'Brien**, Senior Program Coordinator, Utah Physicians for a Healthy Environment, Salt Lake City, Utah

For Brandi, a typical day in her role includes coordinating air purifier orders for K-12 schools and early education centers in Utah. During the pandemic, Brandi's main focus was on improving indoor air quality to encourage a safe and healthy learning environment for Utah's youth. Brandi drew on her passion for equitable learning environments to do this work. When Brandi's not working, she's cheering on the Buffalo Bills or enjoying the plethora of outdoor activities Utah has to offer.

▶   **Caitlin Pedati, MD, MPH, FAAP,** Public Health District Director, Virginia Beach Department of Public Health, Virginia Beach, VA

For Caitlin Pedati, a typical day in her role includes strengthening community partnerships and providing support for the local health department teams in their service to the City of Virginia Beach. During the pandemic, Caitlin's main focus was on assessing current conditions and available information and applying that information to help address the needs of impacted populations, including children in school settings. Caitlin drew on her background as a pediatrician, epidemiologist, and public health professional with experience at the federal, state, and now local levels to do this work. When Caitlin is not working, she likes to spend time with friends and family, and enjoys walks on the beach and cooking new recipes.

▶   **Joanna Pitts, BSN, RN, NCSN, CNOR,** School Health Nurse Consultant, Virginia Department of Health

Joanna collaborates with the Department of Education, the Virginia Chapter of the American Academy of Pediatrics, healthcare providers, parents, schools, and community partners to address various challenges in the school environment. She is passionate about serving her community and works closely with stakeholders to meet the unique needs of K-12 students in Virginia. Together, they aim to eliminate barriers that prevent students from reaching their full potential and to develop innovative solutions that enhance academic performance and success. Recently, Joanna was honored with the Virginia Chapter of the American Academy of Pediatrics Child Advocate Award for 2024. This award recognizes an individual in Virginia who advocates for the rights and welfare of children. Joanna received this recognition for her dedication to making a positive impact on the lives of students and their communities.

▶   **Chris Ralston,** Director III, Facilities Management, Maintenance and Operations, and Resource Management at Sacramento City Unified School District, Sacramento City, California

Chris is in his 21st year of facilities management, his 10th in public education. As facilities director for a school district, Chris is taking the goals set by the superintendent and board in best practices for indoor air quality (IAQ) and making it happen. A good facilities director handles the immediate need and plans for adjustments to them forever, something Sac City has accomplished in its COVID response. Chris has been married for 14 years with two kids.

▶   **Morgan Ripski**, Principal, Champe Carter Consulting, LLC
Morgan Carter Ripski is the principal of Champe Carter Consulting, LLC. She supports schools, nonprofits, and mission-driven leaders at critical inflection points—such as startup or rapid growth—to maximize impact. Previously, she led strategic growth at Collegiate Academies, securing $13M and nine new charters. She also held leadership roles at the Foundation for Science and Math Education and New Schools for New Orleans. Morgan holds degrees from Stanford University and Bates College and lives in New Orleans with her husband and two sons.

▶   **L. Penny Rosenblum, PhD**, Founder, Vision for Independence LLC and Research Professor Emerita University of Arizona, Tucson, Arizona
Through Vision for Independence LLC, Dr. Rosenblum conducts research and designs professional development materials with a focus on children and adults with visual impairments. During the pandemic, Dr. Rosenblum was the director of research at the American Foundation for the Blind and led three national studies that examined the impact of the COVID-19 pandemic on children and adults with visual impairments. The two Access and Engagement studies gathered data from family members, teachers of students with visual impairments, and orientation and mobility specialists. The studies highlighted both the systemic and pandemic-created challenges in educating students with visual impairments, including those with additional disabilities and deafblindness, during the pandemic. With more than 38 years of experience as a teacher of students with visual impairments and a university professor, Dr. Rosenblum drew on her experience with the special education system and her broad network for this work. When Dr. Rosenblum is

not engaged in professional activities, she enjoys bicycling, creating pottery, scrapbooking, traveling, and spending time with her husband and friends.

▶ **Christie Scott, APR,** Director, Board of Education Communications, Montgomery County Board of Education, Montgomery County, Maryland and Former Acting Director, Community Relations, Office of Communications and Community Relations, Fairfax County Public Schools, Virginia

Christie Scott, APR, is a seasoned public relations strategist with over 20 years of experience leading high-impact communications campaigns and building high-performing teams. Known for her innovative approach, she excels at developing strategies that engage communities, build trust, and enhance organizational reputation. Christie has a proven track record of success across diverse sectors, including education, where she led award-winning campaigns such as the VaxUp FCPS initiative. An advocate for the PR profession, she is active in national and regional professional organizations. Christie's leadership continues to inspire organizations nationwide to achieve their communications goals and navigate complex challenges.

▶ **Heidi Schumacher, MD,** Assistant Professor of Pediatrics, University of Vermont Larner College of Medicine and Former Assistant Superintendent, Health and Wellness, Office of the State Superintendent of Education (OSSE), Washington, DC

During the pandemic, a typical day in Heidi's role included issuing school health policy and resources, monitoring compliance and outcomes data, and supporting strategy related to the health and well-being of DC's school and child care communities. During the pandemic, Heidi's main focus was on high quality COVID-19 guidance for educational communities and standing up related implementation supports, including in-school COVID-19 testing and clinical support services. Heidi drew on her training as a pediatrician and experience in federal, state, and local health policy to inform this work. When Heidi's not working, she spends time with her family, including two small children.

► **Christina Silcox, PhD**, Research Director for Digital Health at the Duke-Margolis Center for Health Policy, Washington, DC

Christina Silcox is the research director for Digital Health at the Duke-Margolis Center for Health Policy, working on policy solutions to advance innovation in health and health care and improve regulation, reimbursement, and long-term evaluation of medical products, with a focus on medical devices. During the COVID-19 pandemic, Dr. Silcox led the Center's work on COVID-19 testing, working on policy issues surrounding strategy, regulation, access, payment, and implementation. Dr. Silcox's portfolio also includes multiple areas in digital health policy and real-world evidence. When Christina is not working, her dog Toby enjoys bossing her around and taking her on long walks where he barks at anything on wheels.

► **Irma Martinez Snopek, JD, MEd**, Chief Policy and Communications Officer, Illinois State Board of Education

For Irma Martinez Snopek, a typical day in her role includes providing strategic advice to the state superintendent of education, liaising with the Governor's Office, legislators, agency's board and leadership, managing stakeholder engagement, and overseeing the agency's messaging and policy positions, especially in times of crisis. During the pandemic, Irma's main focus was on developing guidance for the safe return to in-person instructionand communications strategy to respond to school districts' needs, collaborating with multiple stakeholder groups to proactively respond to the pandemic, and emergency rule-making. Irma drew on her background as a classroom teacher, school district administrator, and attorney to do this work. When Irma's not working, she likes to spend time with her husband and two daughters, train for marathons, watch live music, and travel.

► **Audrey Soglin**, Executive Director (former) Illinois Education Association, Springfield, Illinois

Audrey Soglin is the former executive director of the Illinois Education Association (IEA), the statewide teacher's union that represents 135,000 education employees. Audrey started her career as a teacher in Evanston, Illinois, and taught there for 25 years. Prior to becoming the executive director of the Illinois Education Association, Audrey was the director of teaching and learning for IEA and the executive director of the Consortium for Educational Change, a not-for-profit organization founded by IEA, focused on collaboratively improving student learning and achievement. She is also the president of the Partnership for Resilience, which works to transform and integrate education, health care, and community organizations. Audrey is currently an educational consultant.

▶ **Aníbal Soler, Jr.,** Superintendent, Schenectady City Schools, Schenectady, New York

For Aníbal, a typical day in his role includes leading the Schenectady City School District. During the pandemic, Aníbal's main focus was on keeping schools open and trying to provide children and families a safe and welcoming environment. Aníbal drew on his background and experience as a leader, educator, man of color, and father to do this work. When Aníbal's not working, he enjoys spending time with his family and learning more about educational technology.

▶ **Joel Solomon,** Senior Program Manager, Health and Safety, National Education Association, Washington, DC

In 2021, with the understanding that students' learning conditions are educators' working conditions, the National Education Association established its Health and Safety Program to bring focus, support, and an equity lens to resolving new and long-standing health and safety problems in schools serving students from pre-kindergarten through higher education. Joel is the senior program manager who established and continues to lead the Program. The initiative addresses environmental and occupational health and safety hazards like mold, indoor air quality, and chemical safety; violence prevention and response, including gun violence; and school health topics such as student use of personal devices, accountability for social media companies, sexual and reproductive health, and vaccines, immunizations, and infectious diseases. NEA has 3 million members, affiliated associations in every state, and local affiliates in more than 14,000 communities, making it the largest union in the country.

In addition to providing technical and strategic support to its affiliates, the Program develops and delivers health and safety trainings, produces educational material, advocates for strong federal health and safety laws and regulations, and works in partnership with academic institutions, nonprofit organizations, professional associations, and other unions.

▶ **Daniel Soto, EdD, MPH**, Assistant Professor, Department of Population and Public Health Sciences and Former Project Director, Institute for Health Promotion and Disease Prevention Research, University of Southern California, Keck School of Medicine, Los Angeles, California

Daniel Soto, EdD, MPH, leads research and community projects focused on health disparities. During the pandemic, his work centered on collaborating with the California Department of Education, Los Angeles Department of Public Health, and the Los Angeles Mayor's Innovations Team to develop strategies for reopening schools and community centers safely while reducing COVID-19 spread among vulnerable populations. Drawing from his expertise in community relations, public health research, and evaluation, Dr. Soto played a key role in shaping these initiatives. Outside of work, he enjoys spending time with family, riding bikes, and DJing vinyl records.

▶ **Eva Stone, DNP, APRN**, Manager, District Health, Jefferson County Public Schools, Louisville, Kentucky

For Eva Stone, a typical day in her role includes managing health service for a district with nearly 115,000 students and employees. During the pandemic, Eva's main focus was on district surveillance, contact tracing protocols, student and staff testing, and vaccinations. Eva drew on her background in/experience with public health nursing, school health, and systems leadership to do this work. When Eva is not working, she likes to spend time with her husband, children, and grandson.

▶ **Angela Sullivan, PhD**, Assistant Professor, Department of Health Behavior & Assistant Dean for Student and Academic Services and Former Program Director, COVID Testing and Prevention in Alabama's K-12 Schools, The University of Alabama at Birmingham School of Public Health,

For Angela Sullivan, a typical day as assistant professor in the Department of Health Behavior and assistant dean for Student and Academic Services includes teaching, research, and service related to suicide prevention. Dr. Sullivan's main focus is on student services and enrollment management as well as community assessment and suicide prevention. Dr. Sullivan draws on her time as the Project Director for COVID Testing and Prevention in Alabama's K-12 Schools to aid in demonstrating best practices, communications, and relationship building for the next generation of public health practitioners. When she is not working, she likes to hike, explore new places, and spend time entertaining friends and family.

▶   **Sarah Sutton, MPH**, Director of School Programs (former), Health Commons

For Sarah, a typical day in her role during the pandemic included managing a statewide team of implementation specialists, talking to district leaders about their COVID-19 testing programs, and strategizing with the Washington State departments of health and education. During the pandemic, her main focus was on scaling COVID-19 testing to nearly every school in Washington State. Sarah drew on her background in health communication and program implementation to do this work. When Sarah's not working, she likes to garden, hike, and read historical fiction.

▶   **Jonathan Temte, MD, PhD, MS**, Associate Dean for Public Health and Community Engagement, University of Wisconsin School of Medicine and Public Health, Madison, Wisconsin

Jonathan L. Temte is associate dean for Public Health and Community Engagement at the University of Wisconsin School of Medicine and Public Health where he also serves as professor of Family Medicine and Community Health. Dr. Temte has served as the chair of the US Advisory Committee on Immunization Practices and currently chairs the Wisconsin Council on Immunization Practices. He practices and teaches at Wingra Family Medical Center. Dr. Temte has a long history of building bridges between public health and clinical medicine and is the principal investigator of the Oregon Child Absenteeism due to Respiratory Disease Study (ORCHARDS).

▶ **Mary C. Wall, Ed.LD**, Deputy Assistant Secretary for P-12 Education, US Department of Education, 2023-2025; Senior Advisor and Chief of Staff for the Federal COVID-19 Response, The White House, 2021–2023; Chief of Staff, New York City Department of Education, 2020–2021

Dr. Mary C. Wall is a nationally recognized education leader with deep expertise in policy, strategy, and implementation. She recently served as deputy assistant secretary for P-12 Education at the US Department of Education, leading policy and implementation for the Biden-Harris Administration's historic investments in K-12 schools and school-based mental health. Previously, she was chief of staff for both the White House COVID-19 Response Team and the New York City Department of Education, where she led K-12 school reopening efforts from COVID-19 federally and across the nation's largest school district. A Massachusetts native, Mary also served in Boston Public Schools and in the Obama-Biden White House. She holds a bachelor's degree from Boston College and a doctorate in education leadership from Harvard University.

▶ **Rhiannon C. Walker, CNA**, Outreach Medical Assistant, Whiteriver Indian Hospital and Former Nurse, Whiteriver Unified School District Whiteriver, AZ

During the pandemic, Rhiannon was a nurse with the Whiteriver Unified School District. Her main focus during that time was on COVID-19 testing. Rhiannon drew on her background experience with nursing to do this work. When Rhiannon's not working, she likes to attend her children's sports activities that consist of football, baseball, and basketball games and practices. Rhiannon is currently in school to obtain a bachelor's degree in health science and is currently working as an Outreach Medical Assistant at Whiteriver Indian Hospital.

▶ **Katherine H. Walsh**, Assistant Director of Planning, Engineering, Sustainability, and Environment and former Sustainability, Energy, and Environment Program Director, Boston Public Schools, Massachusetts

Serving on the Boston Public Schools Facilities Management leadership team, Katherine manages the Planning, Engineering,

Sustainability, and Environment Division. The team prioritizes critical and equitable operations, maintenance, and districtwide initiatives that improve the sustainability measures and environmental health of all BPS buildings and schoolyards. BPS received the 2023 US Department of Education Green Ribbon School District Sustainability Award. Prior to BPS, Katherine directed The Green Initiative Fund and Student Environmental Resource Center at the University of California, Berkeley. A proud BPS and Boston College graduate, Katherine is committed to bold imagination, climate justice and action, and youth leadership.

▶ **Brian Wegley, PhD**, Superintendent of Schools, Retired, Glenview Northbrook District 30, City of Northbrook and Glenview, Illinois, and Leader, Glenview-Northbrook Coronavirus Response Task Force

Dr. Brian K. Wegley has over 35 years of experience in public education as a physics teacher, associate principal of Curriculum and Instruction and principal at Glenbrook South High School, and as the Superintendent of Northbrook/Glenview School District 30. As superintendent, Brian led a dynamic and cohesive leadership team and board, implemented a strategic vision for long-term educational success, and spearheaded a bond referendum that significantly enhanced school infrastructure.

For Dr. Brian Wegley, a typical day in his role included supporting District 30's administrative team as they managed daily operations and moved forward on their strategic plan. During the pandemic, Brian's main focus was on keeping students at the center of their decision-making efforts and their community united in their response. Brian drew on his experience building and supporting strong teams that focus on strategic objectives. When Brian's not working, he embraces time with his family, enjoying the outdoors with his wife, Kathy, and connecting with his grandson, Henry.

▶ **Laurel L. Williams, DO**, Medical Director of the Centralized Operational Support Hub (COSH), Texas Child Mental Health Care Consortium (TCMHCC), Houston, Texas

For Dr. Williams, a typical day includes overseeing the work of the 12 Child and Adolescent Psychiatry Access Program Hubs (CPAN) and the 12 Texas Child Health Access Thru Telemedicine Hubs (TCHATT) across the Texas. Dr. Williams' main focus has been on developing the standards related to these two population-level programs and assisting in their implementation statewide. Dr. Williams drew on her experience as a clinical leader within Baylor College of Medicine in designing programming that both educates physicians and directly provides services to youth and their families with mental health disorders. When Laurel is not working, she loves to be with her daughter and their menagerie reading, playing tennis, and spending time together.

▶   **Anne Wyllie, PhD**, Global Medical Affairs Lead, Pediatric Pneumococcal Vaccines at Pfizer, Founder, SalivaDirect and Former Research Scientist in Epidemiology, Yale School of Public Health

Anne Wyllie, Ph.D., is the Global Medical Affairs Lead for Pediatric Pneumococcal Vaccines at Pfizer. Formerly a Principal Investigator at Yale School of Public Health, she is internationally recognized for validating and optimizing the use of saliva as a reliable, low-cost sample type for the detection of respiratory pathogens. During the COVID-19 pandemic, she led the development of SalivaDirect, an open-source qPCR protocol that enabled equitable and scalable SARS-CoV-2 testing worldwide. She remains committed to advancing pathogen surveillance, expanding access to low-cost diagnostic tools, and supporting vaccination strategies that strengthen public health. Wyllie earned her PhD from UMC Utrecht and her BSc and MSc from the University of Auckland.

▶   **Kanecia Obie Zimmermann, MD, PhD, MPH**, Associate Professor of Pediatrics, Duke University/Duke Clinical Research Institute, Durham, North Carolina

For Dr. Zimmerman, a typical day in her role includes research in pharmacology clinical trials for children or taking care of children in the intensive care unit. During the pandemic, Dr. Zimmerman's main focus was on collaborating with schools and school districts across the country to better understand mitigation strategies for safe return to K-12 schools. Dr. Zimmerman drew on her background in/experience with patient and family engagement, epidemiology, and running large research programs to do this work. When Dr. Zimmerman's not working, she likes to hang out with her family and watch her children play basketball.

▶ **John Zurbuchen**, Assistant Superintendent at Davis School District, Farmington, Utah

For John, a typical day in his role includes oversight of special education, student & family services, human resources, foundation, and safety and security. During the pandemic, John's main focus was on functioning as the point person for the district's COVID-19 response. John drew on his experience in health care (wife and two daughters are all MD) and Davis County Health Department to do this work. When John's not working, he likes to play in a band, exercise, and travel.

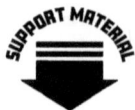

Appendix B: Teaching Guide for this Book

In this teaching guide, we first present discussion questions for each chapter. We then offer hands-on exercises aligned to Chapters 2 through 4. Students can complete these independently or in small groups. Finally, we include a tabletop role-playing exercise that can be completed as a whole class. This exercise draws on concepts across the book.

▶ DISCUSSION QUESTIONS

Chapter 1: Introduction: The Importance of Partnerships in Times of Crises

1. Do you remember the first time you realized COVID-19 would affect your workplace? Was it a gradual growth of concern, or was it immediate? What was your role in your school or organization? Were you responsible for leading your school, district, or organization response?
2. What does partnership mean to you? What partnerships have you been involved with, and how would you characterize them? To what degree were trust, equity, and communication central to your previous partnerships?

Chapter 2: Building and Maintaining Trust

1. K-12 and public health leaders worked together to implement testing and vaccination programs in schools and districts. In what ways did they need to trust each other to do so?
2. How did trust relate to leadership responses to testing and vaccine hesitancy?
3. Each partnership looked to different trusted messengers to engage students, families, and communities in their

pandemic response. What similarities and differences do you see in who these messengers are? Who would serve as trusted messengers in your context?

4. Our case study, Birmingham Public Schools, involves a situation where trust was lost and needed to be rebuilt. What strategies were effective at rebuilding lost trust?

5. One of the key components of trust is respect, which includes respecting differences. What types of differences led to loss of trust? From your perspective, are there differences that K-12 and public health leaders should not accept or respect?

6. Both personal connections and use of data were identified in the chapter as important components of trust. How might these be used to support each other? How might they interfere with each other?

Chapter 3: Planning from the Margins

1. How did K-12 and public health partnerships forged in the pandemic address equity in school populations?

2. How did different districts identify the needs of marginalized populations? What different sources of data did they use?

3. Many districts developed different approaches to prioritization when resources were scarce. What were some of these different approaches?

4. In some districts, "equity" is not valued as a concept. How would you explain the value of an equity lens to those who consider it discrimination?

5. Having a community of practice was an important support for our case study, Jefferson County Public Schools. In what ways did external partnerships support district work, in general and specifically around equity?

Chapter 4: Communicating Clearly in Chaotic Times

1. K-12 and public health leaders had to establish and maintain ongoing coordinated communication to reopen schools. How did different partners approach

this coordination? What are some of the strengths and challenges of different approaches?

2. Trusted messengers are a key component to public health communication. How did different organizations identify the right combination of messenger and message for communities?

3. We discuss the importance of multidirectional communication in this chapter. Explain this concept and why it is critical for K-12 districts.

4. Coordinated communication requires transparency and data sharing. What do these concepts mean, and how did different partnerships address them? What barriers might exist to this type of communication?

Chapter 5: Preparing Leaders for What the Future Brings

1. This book focused on partnerships with public health, but schools serve many functions within a community beyond education and health. What other types of organizations do school districts partner with?

2. The COVID-19 response was an example of crisis leadership. What other school crises exist, and how might the lessons from this book apply to them?

3. In this chapter, we discuss the importance of maintaining partnerships after a crisis. Why is this important, and what mechanisms can be used to do so?

▶ HANDS-ON EXERCISES

Chapter 2: Building and Maintaining Trust

A. Think about a trusting relationship you have with an individual you know in a professional context (e.g., a teacher, an administrator, a community leader). Why do you trust them?

B. Think about a time you lost trust in an individual. What happened?

C. Think about the organization you work for. How do you know that stakeholders trust your organization? Are there any stakeholder groups that do not trust your organization?

D. Make a list of current and potential partners of your organization. For each, how would you assess the current degree of trust, and what steps could you take to increase trust?

E. What is your positionality? How does that inform how you understand different issues and how others perceive you?

F. Imagine your organization is developing a partnership with a new organization. Develop a script you can use when you are introducing yourself to this new potential partner that highlights attributes of relational trust. Then, practice this script with a partner.

Chapter 3: Planning from the Margins

A. Who is "on the margins" in your district? How do you identify marginalized populations, and how do they identify themselves?

B. Listening is a key component to centering equity. What opportunities does your district have for listening to different populations (for example, surveys, group discussions, focus groups, town halls)? To what degree are these opportunities accessible to community members on the margins?

C. Imagine that three classrooms in your school building have old-style chalkboards and every other classroom has whiteboards. Develop a script you can use to explain why those three classrooms will be upgraded to smartboards, but no changes will be made to the other classrooms. Then, practice this script with a partner.

D. Look at the graph below. Which schools would you choose to prioritize to host a vaccination event? What other challenges are those schools struggling with, and how might you take those into account as you plan your events?

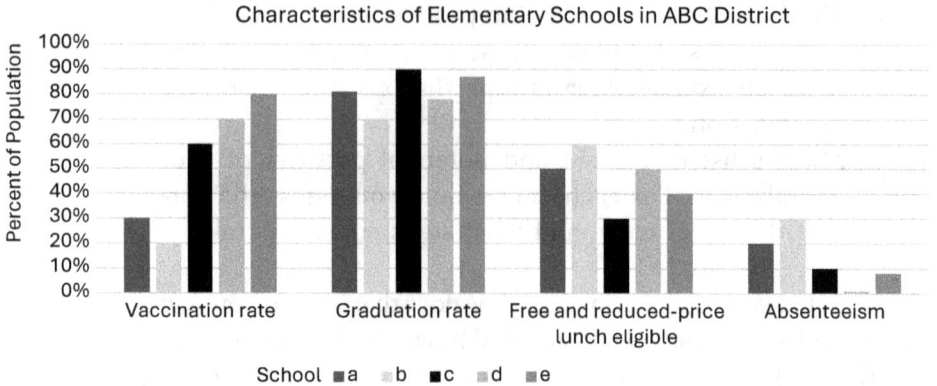

Characteristics of Elementary Schools in ABC District

School ■ a ■ b ■ c ■ d ■ e

E Now look at this graph. In what ways is this school doing better than the district overall? Where is it struggling?

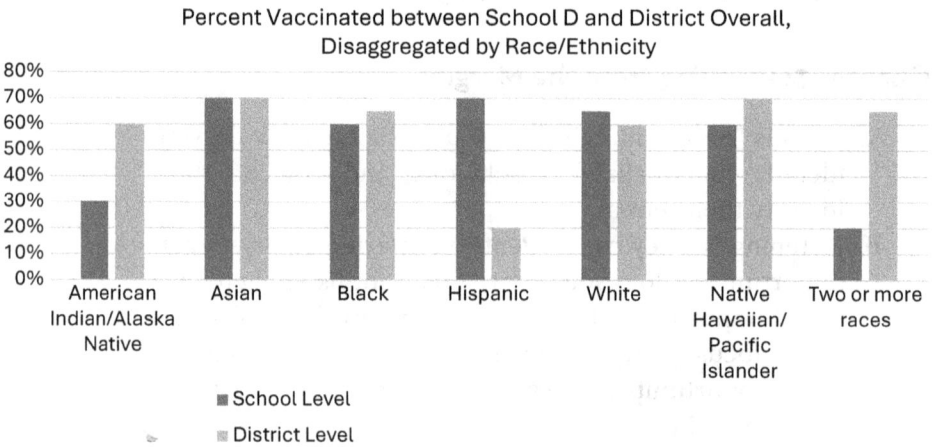

Percent Vaccinated between School D and District Overall, Disaggregated by Race/Ethnicity

■ School Level
■ District Level

F. Use the worksheet available through the book's online resources to make graphs for your own school and district, using the data points given or data points of interest to you. What patterns do you see? What are areas of strength and areas of concern?

Please note that the worksheet is available through the book's online resources

http://www.routledge.com/9781041002383

Chapter 4: Communicating Clearly in Chaotic Times

A. What are current strengths and challenges in communications between different stakeholder groups in your school or district?
   a. What approaches have been tried to support communication? To what degree do you believe them to be successful?
B. Research your district's translation department. How many languages are spoken in your district, and what types of translation services exist? How are messages communicated to parents who speak languages other than English?
C. Identify recent communications that your organization has sent out. Assess their readability in terms of difficulty of text, images, and organization. Would you make any recommendations to make communications more accessible to all stakeholder groups?
D. Imagine that you need to close school for a day (or switch to remote learning) for a personnel reason that cannot be communicated to parents. Develop a script you can use to communicate this to parents. Then, practice this script with a partner.
E. Imagine that your school has partnered with a local nonprofit organization to provide school supplies to students. However, the nonprofit has a religious mission and it wants to provide religious books along with notebooks, pencils, and other supplies. Develop a script you can use when you need to ask the nonprofit to not include these books. Then, practice this script with a partner.

▶ TABLETOP ROLEPLAY EXERCISE

Tabletop roleplay is a traditional learning activity within public health and emergency management, in which participants attempt to solve a challenge that the organization might face by taking on roles of different individuals within the organization.

Purpose

- Understand a complex situation from different perspectives.
- Explore how partnerships can work in action.
- Develop skills in problem-solving and partnership work.

Background

This exercise takes place in a small K-12 school district, with approximately 200 students per grade. There is one hospital system in town, offering primarily urgent care support.

Roles

Each of these participants should participate in this activity; if all are not able to participate, prioritize the starred roles. If more than ten participants are available, individuals can partner up on roles. In addition, one person will take on the role of the facilitator of the exercise, typically the course instructor. The facilitator should read through the entire exercise before beginning the roleplay.

1. District superintendent or appointee
2. District nursing lead*
3. Elementary school principal*
4. Elementary school nurse*
5. Elementary school secretary
6. Public health director*
7. Public health communication lead
8. PTA president*
9. School board president*
10. Hospital system emergency manager*

Facilitator Reads the Scenario

The local hospital system has informed the public health director that there have been a large number of elementary school–aged children coming in with varying degrees of respiratory illness. Many have tested positive for influenza A.

Questions to Ask

- Public health director, what would you like to do?
  - o Who needs to be contacted?
  - o What response is needed from your side?
  - o What resources are required?

Have public health director call the school principal and role-play the initial conversation. Possible outcomes:

- What are the goals of the school and the public health department?
- Discuss a communication plan. Have them develop a communication plan with their team.
  - o Distribute communication plan to PTA president and school board president and have them react
- Request data.
  - o Attendance data by grade (see school demographics table)
  - o School demographics and vaccination rates (see school demographics table)
- Other outcomes, as determined by the conversation

Set up a meeting with each of the participants. Have them role-play the meeting after the facilitator reads the following update.
School records show that the next day, 20% of students are absent from the elementary school, with additional absences from the middle school and high school. Additionally, six teachers are out (either sick themselves or caring for their own sick children).

- What are the goals of the school, the school district, the hospital system, and the public health department?
- What response is needed from each side?
- What resources are required?
- Who is going to be in charge of each piece?

At this point, you should be able to allow the discussion and planning to continue with limited guidance. If there is a lull in conversation, or there is confusion, use the following questions to focus the discussion.

Probing Questions to Ask:

- Public health director, what would you like to do now?
  o Will you work through the school or independently or both?
  o Who else needs to be involved?
- School principal and superintendent, what would you like to do now?
  o Who on your team is going to lead this response?
  o What and how will you communicate?
    ▪ With staff
    ▪ With families
  o What considerations do you have to make about equity?
  o Will you need to set up distance learning, and, if so, how will you do that?
- School nurse and district nursing lead, what do you need?
  o Do you want to be involved in communication?
  o Do you want support from public health?
- School secretary, what is your role?
  o What will you be saying to families who call to report an absence?
  o Will you be looking into the data? What will you look for?
- PTA president, what will your response be?
  o Are there trust issues to navigate?
  o Do you want/need to be involved in communication?
- School board president, what is your role?
  o Which of the pillars of partnership (trust, equity, communication) may be weakest in your district? What will you do about it?
  o What policies and procedures are in place?
- Hospital emergency manager, what is your role?
  o Do you need to build communication pathways with the school?
  o What policies and procedures are in place?

- All
  - o What do the data show?
    - Are there particular groups most affected?
    - Are there demographic changes to be aware of?
    - Do you notice any patterns of concern?
  - o What sort of relationship is needed here?
    - Who is in charge of what?
    - What are the components of your response, and who needs to be involved in each?
    - Who isn't at the table?
  - o What are the trust issues to consider?
  - o What are the equity issues to consider?
  - o What are the communication issues to consider?

Potential data for school districts

Attendance records by school over a 2-week period in February

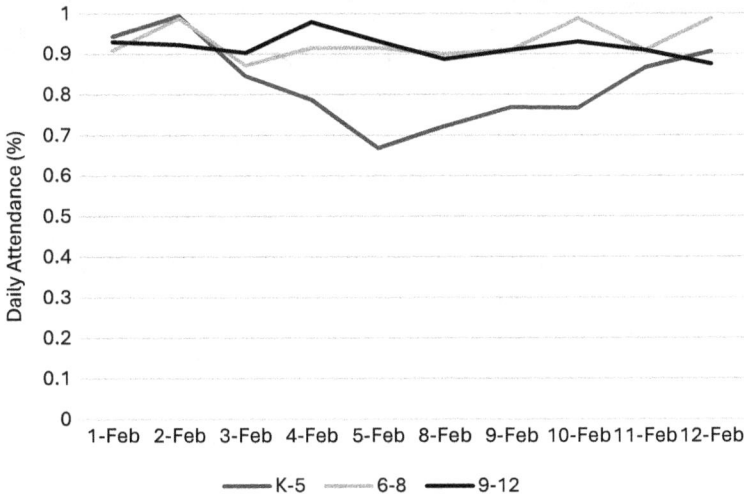

▶ SCHOOL DEMOGRAPHICS

	Vaccinated	Low-Income	K-5	6-8	9-12
White	79%	52%	65%	66%	67%
Black	82%	62%	33%	30%	30%
Other	76%	48%	3%	4%	4%
Hispanic	64%	72%	42%	30%	25%

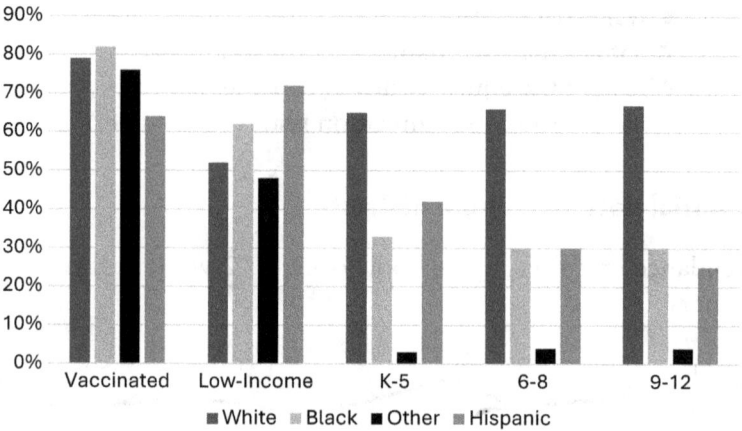

■White ■Black ■Other ■Hispanic

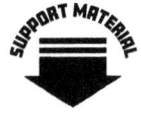

Appendix C: Additional Resources

▶ **PROTOCOLS FOR IDENTIFYING, DEVELOPING, AND STRENGTHENING PARTNERSHIPS**

- How to Build Cross-Sector Partnerships That Improve Public Health, 2024. Public Health Communications Collaborative. Available at https://publichealthcollaborative. org/communication-tools/how-to-build-cross-sector-partnerships-that-improve-public-health/
- Building Non-Traditional Public Health Multisector Partnerships: How State and Territorial health Agencies Can Leverage Healthy People 2030 for Innovative Collaboration to Improve Health Outcomes and Advance Health Equity, 2025. Available at https://www.astho.org/49009e/ globalassets/toolkit/building-non-traditional-public-health-multisector-partnerships.pdf
- The Secret to Successful Health Partnerships, 2015, by Lawrence Prybil, Robert Pestronk, Paul Jarris, and Rich Umbdenstock with the Robert Wood Johnson Foundation. Available at https://www.rwjf.org/en/general-library-listing. html?k=&s=0&rpg=15&ff=topics,initiatives,content-types,authors,health-factors&a=authors:LPrybil
- Recommendations for Strengthening Partnerships Between Health Departments and Community-Based Organizations, 2024, by Asma Day and Francesca Hill with the CDC Foundation. Available at https://www.cdcfoundation. org/blog/new-tool-strengthening-partnerships-between-health-departments-and-communities
- Partnership Self-Assessment Tool – Questionnaire, 2002, by Center for the Advancement of Collaborative Strategies in Health. Available at https://hdl.handle.net/10214/3129
- Principles of Partnership Self-Assessment Tool, 2020, by Greater Plains Collaborative Clinical Research network.

Available at https://www.pcori.org/sites/default/files/3894_GPC_Principles-Partnership-Self-Assessment.pdf

▶ COMMUNICATING SCIENCE TO THE GENERAL PUBLIC

- National Center for Science Education classroom resources https://ncse.ngo/supporting-teachers/classroom-resources
- AAAS resource center on Science Education. Available at https://www.aaas.org/focus-areas/science-education
- National Science Teachers Association case studies. Available at https://www.nsta.org/case-studies
- Smithsonian Institute Learning Lab. Available at https://learninglab.si.edu/
- Genetics teaching resources. Available at https://learn.genetics.utah.edu/
- Fred Hutch Cancer Center SciEd program. Available at https://www.fredhutch.org/en/education-training/about-science-education.html
- Your Local Epidemiologist substack, "Providing a direct line of" translated "public health science to you," available at https://yourlocalepidemiologist.substack.com/
- CDC's Crisis & Emergency Risk Communication (CERC) Manual, 2024. Available at https://www.cdc.gov/cerc/php/cerc-manual/index.html

▶ ADDRESSING INACCURATE HEALTH INFORMATION

- Practical Playbook for Addressing Health Rumors: A Helpful Tool for Practitioners, 2024. Center for Health Security, John Hopkins Bloomberg School of Public Health. Available at https://centerforhealthsecurity.org/sites/default/files/2024-07/24-07-cdc-misinfo-playbook-v2.pdf
- Health Misinformation, 2025. Office of the Surgeon General, U.S. Department of Health and Human Services. Available at https://www.hhs.gov/surgeongeneral/reports-and-publications/health-misinformation/index.html

- A Community Toolkit for Addressing Health Misinformation: Information that is false, inaccurate, or misleading according to the best available evidence of the time, 2021. U.S. Department of Health and Human Services. Available at https://www.hhs.gov/sites/default/files/health-misinformation-toolkit-english.pdf

▶ EXAMPLES OF CLEAR PUBLIC HEALTH RESPONSE GUIDANCE

- COVID-19, 2025. Washington State Department of Health. Available at https://doh.wa.gov/emergencies/covid-19
- COVID-19: Protect Yourself & Others, 2024. Minnesota Department of Health. Available at https://www.health.state.mn.us/diseases/coronavirus/prevention.html
- COVID-19 Testing in K-12 Settings: A Playbook for Educators and Leaders, 2021. The Rockefeller Foundation. Available at https://www.rockefellerfoundation.org/wp-content/uploads/2021/02/The-RockefellerFoundation-Covid-19-K-12-Testing-Playbook-for-Educators-and-Leaders.pdf
- Supporting Student Health and Wellness During Public Health Emergencies, 2024. American Academy of Pediatrics. Available at https://www.aap.org/en/patient-care/school-health/supporting-student-health-and-wellness-during-public-health-emergencies/
- Pandemic Plan, 2020. Suffolk County Schools. Available at https://resources.finalsite.net/images/v1583427132/suffield/dyk3y4ucdnucgj3r0pti/PANDEMICPLANFebruary2020.pdf

▶ K-12 EMERGENCY PREPAREDNESS GUIDES

- Guide for Developing High-Quality School Emergency Operations Plans, 2013. FEMA, U.S. Department of Education. Available at https://rems.ed.gov/docs/School_Guide_508C.pdf
- Database of Publicly Available Publications and Guidance Documents from the Readiness and Emergency

management for Schools (REMS) Technical Assistance Center. Available at https://rems.ed.gov/REMSPublications.aspx

▶ ASSET MAPPING AND NEEDS ASSESSMENT TOOLS

- Community Assessments: Three Examples of Asset-Oriented Assessment Tools. (2017). Oklahoma State University Extension. https://extension.okstate.edu/fact-sheets/community-assessments-three-examples-of-asset-oriented-assessment-tools.html
- Conducting Rural Health Research, Needs Assessments, and Program Evaluations. (2024). Rural Health Information Hub. https://www.ruralhealthinfo.org/topics/rural-health-research-assessment-evaluation
- Asset-Based Community Development Workbooks and Guides. (2025). Asset-Based Community Development Institute. https://www.abcdinstitute.org/content.aspx?page_id=22&club_id=104994&module_id=683173
- School Health Index. (2025). Action for Healthy Kids. https://www.actionforhealthykids.org/school-health-index/

▶ PRIORITY SETTING TOOLS

- Guide to Prioritization Techniques. National Association of County and City Health Officials. https://www.naccho.org/uploads/downloadable-resources/Gudie-to-Prioritization-Techniques.pdf
- Priority Setting and Decision-Making Framework Toolkit. (2010). National Collaborating Centre for Methods and Tools. https://www.nccmt.ca/knowledge-repositories/search/353

▶ EQUITY AUDIT TOOLS

- *Equity Audits: A Practical Leadership Tool for Developing Equitable and Excellent Schools* (2009). Linda Skrla,

Kathryn Bell McKenzie James Joseph Scheurich, eds.. Thousand Oaks, CA: Corwin Press.

- How to Conduct a Systemic Equity Audit. Edutopia. (2024). https://www.edutopia.org/article/conducting-school-wide-equity-audit/
- Resource Equity Diagnostics for Districts. Alliance for Resource Equity. https://educationresourceequity.org/wp-content/uploads/documents/diagnostic.pdf
- Criteria for an Equitable School – Equity Audit. Mid-Atlantic Equity Consortium. (2020). https://maec.org/wp-content/uploads/2016/04/Criteria-for-an-Equitable-School-2020-accessible.pdf

▶ HISTORY OF PUBLIC HEALTH IN THE UNITED STATES

- *The Future of Public Health*, 1988. Institute of Medicine (US) Committee for the Study of the Future of Public Health. Washington (DC): National Academies Press
- *The Great Influenza: The Story of the Deadliest Pandemic in History*, 2020. John Barry. United Kingdom: Penguin Press.
- *Maladies of Empire*, 2020. Jim Downs. Cambridge, MA: Harvard University Press.
- *Typhoid Mary: Captive to the Public's Health*, 1997. Judith Walzer Leavitt. Beacon Press.

▶ HISTORY OF NATIVE AMERICAN BOARDING SCHOOLS

1. *Boarding School Seasons: American Indian Families 1900–1940*. Brenda Childs. Lincoln, Nebraska: University of Nebraska Press.
2. *Education for extinction, 1995*. David Wallace Adams. Lawrence: University Press of Kansas
3. *Researching My Heritage: The Old Leupp Boarding School Historic Site*, 2021. Daniel Two Bears. *kiva*, *87*(3), 336–353.

4. *Stringing Rosaries: The History, the Unforgivable, and the Healing of Northern Plains American Indian Boarding School Survivors, 2019.* Denise K. Lajimodiere. Fargo, NDÑ North Dakota State University Press
5. *They Called it Prairie Light: The Story of Chilocco Indian School*, 1995. K. Tsianina Lomawaima. Lincoln, Nebraska: University of Nebraska Press.

▶ HISTORY OF MEDICAL MISTREATMENT OF MINORITIZED AMERICANS

- About the USPHS Syphilis Study. (2025). Tuskegee University. Available from https://www.tuskegee.edu/about-us/centers-of-excellence/bioethics-center/about-the-usphs-syphilis-study
- *Medical apartheid: The dark history of medical experimentation on Black Americans from colonial times to the present*, 2006. Harriet A. Washington. Doubleday Books.
- *Where Biology Ends and Bias Begins: Lessons on Belonging from Our DNA*, 2025. Shoumita Dasgupta. University of California Press.
- Racism and Child Health, 2025, Mary T Bassett, Zinzi Bailey, and Aletha Maybank. In Nelson's *Textbook of Pediatrics*, edited by Robert Kliegman. Elsevier.
- *Building the Worlds that Kill Us: Disease, Death, and Inequality in American* History, 2026. David Rosner and Gerald Markowitz, Columbia University Press.

Appendix D: Commonly Used Abbreviations in the Book

Abbreviation	Definition
ADHS	Arizona Department of Health Services
AFCEMA	Atlanta-Fulton County Emergency Management Agency
ASHRAE	American Society of Heating, Refrigerating, and Air-Conditioning Engineers
BPS	Boston Public Schools
CCLG	Cross-City Learning Group
CDC	Centers for Disease Control and Prevention
CDPH	Chicago Department of Public Health
CLIA	Clinical Laboratory Improvement Amendments
CLS	Chief Leschi Schools
COP	Communities of Practice
CPS	Chicago Public Schools
EPA	Environmental Protection Agency
ESSER	Elementary and Secondary School Emergency Relief Fund
FCS	Fulton County Board of Public Health
FERPA	Family Educational Rights and Privacy Act
HIPAA	Health Insurance Portability and Accountability Act of 1996
IAQ	Indoor Air Quality
JCPS	Jefferson County Public Schools
K-12	Kindergarten to grade 12 schools
NSPRA	National School Public Relations Association
ORCHARDS	Oregon Child Absenteeism Due to Respiratory Disease Study
OSD	Oregon School District

PREP Act	Public Readiness and Emergency Preparedness Act
RSV	Respiratory Syncytial Virus
SLV	School-located vaccination
TCS	Tribally controlled schools
UAB	The School of Public Health at the University of Alabama, Birmingham
UIUC	University of Illinois Urbana-Champaign
UW	University of Wisconsin
VDH	Virginia Department of Health
WHO	World Health Organization
FDA	U.S. Food and Drug Administration

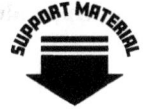

Appendix E: Tips for a Community Survey

▶ **BEFORE STARTING A SURVEY, YOU SHOULD MAKE THE FOLLOWING CLEAR**

- What is the population you want answers from?
- What information do you want to know?
- What additional information would help you interpret results?

Once you have laid out the purpose of the survey, you can start to design it. Following are some general suggestions for designing the overall questionnaire and for designing individual questions.

▶ **GENERAL TIPS FOR SURVEY QUESTIONNAIRE DEVELOPMENT**

- *Introduction*: It can be helpful to start with a brief introduction, so people will know what to expect. It can include the purpose of the survey and how long it will take.
- *Instructions*: This can guide people who are not used to taking surveys.
- *Question Grouping*: Make it easy to get through the survey by allowing people to focus on one topic at a time. Use a grouping mechanism that makes sense.
- *Question Order*: The most important questions should go first, in case people drop out.
- *Length*: Shorter is better!
- *Language*: If you need to include multiple languages, be sure to have a good translator rewrite the questions.
- *Accessibility*: Be aware of the needs of your community and choose a survey method and mode that is accessible to most.

▶ GENERAL TIPS FOR QUESTION DEVELOPMENT

- multiple choice questions are more likely to be answered and easier to analyze than open-ended or fill in the blank, for example.
- be precise.
- don't combine multiple questions—one idea per question.
- don't "lead"—ask the question as objectively as possible.
- use the language your community would understand.
- ask questions your community can answer easily.
- be clear if you want an opinion or a fact.
- avoid words like always or never.

▶ SURVEY ANALYSIS

So you have responses—great! Now what do you do?

1. Check your representation. Do survey respondents represent the population you want answers from?
2. Look at the main question.
3. Look at variation around the main question. Do the responses to the main question differ among different demographic groups?
4. Repeat steps 2 and 3 for any secondary questions.
5. What does it mean and how will you act? Go back to your survey respondents and share the results. Ask them to help with interpreting what it all means. Don't do a survey for the sake of doing a survey—it should lead to action! Use the survey results and engagement with your survey respondents to guide you.

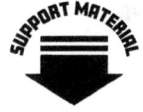

Appendix F: Thinking About Creating a Dashboard? Start Here

Data dashboards can help schools and public health partners share key information with different audiences in one easy-to-access place. When updated regularly and designed with users' needs in mind, dashboards promote transparency—and help families, staff, and partners understand what's happening and why certain decisions are being made.

If you are planning to build a dashboard to inform school communities during a public health crisis—or even to support coordination behind the scenes—start with a plan. These questions can help. We've included example answers to show how this might look in practice.

1. What is the purpose of the dashboard?
   What do you want this tool to show or support?

   - Track health-related absences across schools.
   - Display air quality levels and related school closures.
   - Share updates on student wellness screenings or chronic condition management.
   - Show availability and hours for school-based health resources (e.g., clinics, counseling, testing).

2. Who is the intended audience?
   How can you make it clear, usable, and accessible for that group?

   - Families, including those with limited digital access.
   - School staff and administrators.
   - Public health partners.
   - Community organizations.

   a. **Is the language appropriate for the audience?**

      - Remove jargon (e.g., use "breathing problems" instead of "respiratory distress").

- Write in plain language, aiming for middle-school reading level.

b. Are all languages spoken in your community represented?

- Offer dashboards in languages spoken by your families.
- Review translations with local bilingual family liaisons.

c. Are visual elements accessible?

- Use colorblind-friendly palettes.
- Add alt-text to describe any graphics or visuals.
- Ensure screen-reader compatibility (A screen reader is assistive technology that helps people who are blind or have low vision use computers, phones, and other digital devices. It reads aloud the text on the screen or sends the content to a refreshable braille display. Screen readers also describe menus, buttons, links, and images (if they have alt text), so users can navigate websites, apps, and documents).

3. What data are available?
   How reliable and up to date is the information you'll share?

   - Nurse visits by reason or trend.
   - School-level air quality readings.
   - Community vaccination rates or access to health services.

   a. Are there privacy concerns?

   - Mask any small group data to protect student identity. For example, if there are only three Asian American students, do not report out data on that group.
   - Avoid identifying individuals by health condition or location.

   b. How frequently will the data be updated?

   - Daily health office logs summarized weekly.
   - Real-time updates for closures or health alerts.

4. Where will the dashboard live?
How will people find it?

  - Linked on the district website or family portal.
  - Shared in newsletters and parent apps.
  - Embedded in principal updates or school health pages.

5. Who will create the dashboard?
Do you have the right people and tools to build it?

  - A school IT/data team working with local health department analysts.
  - Support from external vendors using tools like Google Looker, Tableau, or Power BI.

a. What approvals are needed?

  - District communications or legal team review.
  - Accessibility and translation review.
  - Superintendent or board sign-off for public release.

6. How will you roll out the dashboard?
How will people learn about it and give feedback?

a. How will you publicize it?

  - Announce at back-to-school nights or town halls.
  - Share links through email, text, and social media.
  - Highlight through trusted messengers like principals or school nurses.

b. How will you know if it's being used?

  - Monitor traffic using analytics.
  - Use QR codes on flyers to track engagement.

c. How will you know if it's working for users?

  - Add a quick survey ("Was this helpful?" or "I would attend a future event like this with a "Yes" or "No" option).
  - Host focus groups with staff and families.

d. How will you respond to questions or concerns?

  - Provide an FAQ section.
  - Offer a contact email or helpline.
  - Partner with community groups to gather feedback.

Index

Pages in *italics* refer to figures.

For Product Safety Concerns and Information please contact our EU
representative GPSR@taylorandfrancis.com
Taylor & Francis Verlag GmbH, Kaufingerstraße 24, 80331 München, Germany

www.ingramcontent.com/pod-product-compliance
Lightning Source LLC
Chambersburg PA
CBHW062023270326
41929CB00014B/2295